Can Survive

Reclaiming Your Life After Cancer

Susan Nessim and Judith Ellis

HOUGHTON MIFFLIN COMPANY

Boston • New York 2000

Library of Congress Cataloging-in-Publication Data
Nessim, Susan.
Can survive : reclaiming your life after cancer / Susan Nessim
and Judith Ellis. — Revised and updated.
    p.   cm.
Revised ed. previously published under the title: Cancervive.
Includes bibliographical references and index.
ISBN 0-618-00417-3
1. Cancer — Patients — Rehabilitation. 2. Cancer —
Psychological aspects. 3. Self-help groups. I. Ellis, Judith.
II. Nessim, Susan. Cancervive. III. Title.
RC262.N476   2000
616.99'403 — dc21   99-058373

This book was originally published in 1991 as *Cancervive:
The Challenge of Life After Cancer.*

Book design by Joyce C. Weston

QUM   10 9 8 7 6 5 4 3 2 1

Contents

Can Survive

For Lisa Jamison and Lenore Ellis

In the depth of winter I finally learned that within
me there lay an invincible summer.

— Albert Camus

Acknowledgments

We want to extend our thanks to the following individuals for their advice and support: Deborah T. Berg, R.N., the Dana Farber Cancer Center; Julie Brennglass, M.F.C.C., Cancervive Social Services Director; attorney at law Timothy Calonita; Grace Christ, L.C.S.W., Columbia University; Barry M. Daste, Ph.D., Louisiana State University; Nancy Davenport-Ennis, director of the National Patient Advocate Foundation; Robert Enteen, Ph.D.; Daniel Fiduccia of Candlelighters Childhood Cancer Foundation; Camilla B. Fore, R.N.; Patricia Ganz, M.D., University of California, Los Angeles; Daniel Green, M.D., Department of Pediatrics, Roswell Park Memorial Institute; attorney at law Barbara Hoffman; Sandra Horning, M.D., Stanford University Medical Center; Ernest Katz, Ph.D., director of behavioral sciences at the Los Angeles Children's Hospital; Frank K. Meyskens, Jr., M.D., director of the Chow Cancer Center at the University of California, Irvine; consumer advocate Ralph Nader; Joe Neglia, M.D., assistant professor of pediatric oncology, University of Minnesota; Christine Perkins, M.F.C.C.; Leslie R. Schover, Ph.D., the M.D. Anderson Cancer Center in Houston, Texas; Les Gallo-Silver, senior social worker at New York University's Medical Center; consumer writer Wesley J. Smith; Jordan Wilbur, M.D.; California Pacific Medical Center, San Francisco.

Our gratitude to editor Rux Martin at Houghton Mifflin,

whose suggestions for improving the manuscript were insightful and invaluable. Appreciation is also extended to Russell Galen at Scovil, Chickak & Galen for his encouragement and perseverance. And a special thanks to ABC correspondent Sam Donaldson for lending his support to this project.

Finally, we wish to express our deep gratitude to the many survivors who took the time and had the courage to share their stories with us. Their contributions gave this book life.

Foreword

FOR MOST OF my life, the word *cancer* was an abstraction. I knew people who had beaten cancer, as well as those who'd succumbed to it. But that was the extent of my experience with the disease, and I certainly didn't give it a lot of thought.

That is, until the summer of 1995. It was then that I discovered an enlarged lymph node in my groin, which was, as it turned out, the legacy of a suspicious-looking mole I'd had removed from my ankle almost eight years before. At that time, three different biopsy results came back negative. But now, a needle biopsy of the enlarged lymph node revealed a different diagnosis: stage-three melanoma.

I knew I had a major fight on my hands, and I immediately presumed it was a fight I had no chance of winning. What I knew about melanoma left me with the impression that it was the Tyrannosaurus rex of cancers. Also, I had grown up during a time when a cancer diagnosis was considered a death sentence, with no chance for appeal. I concluded that at best I had two, maybe three months to live.

My physician suggested I see Dr. Steven Rosenberg, chief surgeon at the National Cancer Institute in Bethesda, Maryland. Dr. Rosenberg, a melanoma specialist who has successfully treated patients with advanced forms of the disease, examined me, my biopsy slides, and CAT-scan results. I waited, braced for the worst. Instead, he told me rather matter-of-factly that I had a good chance of living a long, healthy life. I didn't believe him, and I told him so. But of course I wanted to believe him, and I was willing to listen. As it turns out, I was eligible to be treated at NCI as a research patient. A week later, I underwent surgery there to remove the lymph node, as well as several surrounding nodes.

The day of that initial consultation with Dr. Rosenberg, I assembled my Washington, D.C.–based *PrimeTime Live* staff and informed them of my diagnosis. I told them about the cancer therapy options I was considering, stressing my intention of continuing to work a normal schedule. I wanted no special treatment.

I'm a private person, but it never occurred to me *not* to tell them. It was my responsibility to let them know what was going on. Also, after more than thirty years spent covering Washington, I know that cover-ups don't work. And although I didn't make an active effort at the time to publicize my condition, I realized the news would eventually get out.

That was on a Friday. The following Monday, I was reading all about it in the newspapers and fielding calls from concerned friends and colleagues, some of whom had waged their own battle with cancer. It was then that I discovered the powerful therapeutic effect of talking with other cancer survivors. I heard from former FBI director William Sessions, who had been successfully treated for melanoma while helming the bureau. Senator Connie Mack called to tell me about a melanoma lesion he'd had removed a few years earlier, and how he was now doing fine. I slowly began to realize that there is life after cancer, and it's my intention to make it a productive one.

That is why a book like *Can Survive: Reclaiming Your Life After Cancer* is so important. A cancer diagnosis leaves you feeling sad and scared, overwhelmed and isolated. Treatment can leave you physically devastated. And as so many former cancer patients know, picking up the pieces during and after recovery presents its own set of physical, emotional, and social challenges.

When it comes to dealing with the aftermath of cancer, I've

been fortunate. The only long-term effect of my surgery is chronic swelling in my right leg, which is kept in check through the use of a full-length support stocking. Of course, I think about recurrence now and then—is there a cancer survivor who doesn't? But I keep in mind that I was sixty-one years old when diagnosed with this particular chronic disease, and no one lives forever.

Every now and then I'll hear from a survivor who will tell me how their cancer helped them become a kinder, gentler person. I don't know if that's necessarily been my experience. I have not become the wonderful, loveable person that I never was. I still bark at my assistant from time to time, and I continue to press those tape editors who make a wrong edit. I am not, in short, a case of Saul becoming St. Paul.

However, cancer *has* given me a new sense of mission. I remain acutely aware of and involved in cancer causes and issues and have a better understanding of how advocacy and education serve as important weapons in fighting this disease. And because I am in the public arena, my involvement can help attract attention and rally support to increase funding for cancer research. In fact, it was during my initial involvement with an ABC news special on cancer, hosted by news anchor Peter Jennings and broadcast in 1998, that I was put in touch with Susan Nessim. We discussed her involvement in a segment of the show devoted to cancer survivorship, and it was through her involvement that I learned about the issues her organization addresses.

When *Cancervive,* the first edition of this book, was published in 1991, it was the first work of its kind to examine the special needs and concerns of *recovering* cancer patients. The book offered positive, empathetic advice and authoritative information to help survivors grapple with the many unforeseen and often unavoidable difficulties they encountered, such as how to deal with fears of recurrence, possible long-term side effects of treatment, insurance obstacles, relationship problems, and more.

Since that book's debut, a great deal has changed in the world of cancer treatment, and subsequently, issues involving long-term survivorship. This revised edition updates and expands on information found in the first edition and provides additional testimony through the voices of cancer survivors.

There are ten million cancer survivors alive today — double the number a decade ago — living proof that the tide is turning. With the likes of Dr. Steven Rosenberg and the many other cancer researchers on the front line, it won't be long before we win this war. In the meantime, we need to let the world know that it is possible to have a history of cancer and still enjoy a happy, healthy, forward-looking life. *Can Survive* is a book designed to help pave the way.

— Sam Donaldson
August 1999

Introduction

WHEN I LEFT Stanford University Medical Center twenty-five years ago after treatment for cancer, I wasted no time in charging back into life. My one desire was to put the experience behind me.

But it wasn't long before I discovered that although I was cancer-free, I certainly wasn't free of cancer. A series of personal incidents revealed that there was more to overcoming this disease than surviving the hardships of treatment. Instead, the end of treatment marked the beginning of a new and unexpected challenge: adapting to life after cancer.

Fifteen years ago I started Cancervive, a Los Angeles–based nonprofit organization for recovered cancer patients, because I realized I wasn't alone in the problems I faced. Since then I've heard from thousands of survivors who also find that the struggle against the disease is only half the battle. Although their doctors advise them to get back to work and on with their lives, that isn't always as easy as it sounds.

On leaving the hospital or outpatient clinic, recovering cancer patients are faced with a bumpy transitional period as they learn to adjust to life without the intensive medical support they received throughout treatment. During this particularly vulnerable time, survivors encounter unanticipated difficulties, such as anxiety over ending treatment, delayed stress reactions, fear of recurrence, and a variety of other problems of adjustment that are an inescapable part of living with a chronic, life-threatening disease. In addition, some must learn to adapt to chronic pain or the loss of a body part, while others are at risk for long-term complications of treatment.

As they reenter the mainstream, recovered patients must frequently contend with such formidable cancer-related obstacles as employment and insurance discrimination, altered family relationships, loss of friends, and for some, loss of fertility. In short, cancer creates lifelong physical, emotional, and psychosocial changes. And because there is virtually no comprehensive support system in place for survivors, they are all too often forced to grapple with these changes on their own.

During my recovery, I searched in vain for information that could shed light on the many post-treatment problems I was encountering. Virtually every book on cancer then centered on the immediate needs of patients fighting the disease, emphasizing modes of treatment, techniques for coping, and the issues of death and dying. While these issues are urgent and undeniably important, they aren't always relevant to those who have moved beyond the patient stage. I knew that the needs of survivors, while different, were no less significant.

That, simply put, is the reason for this book.

This new edition updates and expands on the information and resources found in that original survivor's guide. The names of the survivors interviewed for this book have been changed, and several of their stories are composites, drawn from the transcripts of those who shared similar problems. The guarantee of anonymity freed many of them to reveal the profound emotional turmoil that is so much a part of the legacy of cancer. Interwoven with their experiences are the advice and observations of noted authorities, including doctors, oncology nurses, psychologists, and social workers — all experts in the field of cancer survivorship.

The experiences recounted in this book do not always reflect the triumphant, happily-ever-after image of cancer survivors so often presented in the mass media. Life after cancer is rarely as neat and tidy as that. Rather, our stories show how, by working through the aftermath of cancer, survivors can derive new meaning and purpose from the experience and thereby close the circle on their recovery. Life after cancer may be inalterably changed, but in many ways it can also be more vital and rewarding. The stories of many of the survivors told in this book are testament to that reality.

Cancer survivorship is a growing phenomenon in this country. Approximately one million Americans are diagnosed each year with cancer. Of that number, half can expect to live disease-free for five or more years.* It is estimated that by the year 2000, there will be ten million cancer survivors in the U.S., a figure that will continue to increase each year. As a result, the medical community, the media, and even Congress have begun to take notice of the complex array of issues confronting survivors. But despite greater public awareness and education, recovered patients still find that they must pick their way through the psychosocial land mines that dot the field of survivorship.

While this new edition provides many new revisions to the original book, its underlying purpose remains unchanged: to help survivors realize that they are not alone, and that the pain of loss, so inextricably bound to the cancer experience, holds the potential for immeasurable gains and growth.

— Susan Nessim
August 1999

---

*The survival time that is traditionally designated to mean a "cure."

1
My Story as a Survivor

AS THE PLANE MADE its final approach into Pittsburgh, I peered out the window at the mosaic of shimmering lights below. From my aerial viewpoint, I tried to form a first impression of the city I would soon be calling home. The pilot banked hard, and the soft diffusion of city lights suddenly gave way to the night sky. I sat back in my seat, closed my eyes, and focused my thoughts on the days that lay ahead.

With this trip, I felt certain I was finally free of the past and the threat it had once held for me. Four years earlier, in 1975 at the age of seventeen, I had been diagnosed with rhabdomyosarcoma, a rare form of cancer that attacked the soft tissue in my right thigh. With that diagnosis I embarked on a year-long medical odyssey, and learned firsthand what it meant to live with the imminent threat of dying. As grim as the experience was, I emerged from it with new eyes. The world was somehow more vivid to me, richer and more sharply edged. I was exhilarated with the simple joy of being alive and in good health.

But tonight I was also a little scared. I was flying to Pennsylvania to meet my fiancé's parents. As significant as that ritual is for most people, to me it held an even deeper meaning. A commitment to marriage meant a commitment to the future, a personal acknowledgment that I was going to live and thrive. I'd finally put cancer behind me.

Michael, my fiancé, was at the airport waiting to greet me. We had met more than a year before at the University of Colorado–Boulder, shortly after I'd returned to college following cancer treatment. I was then a sophomore intent on getting a degree in business. Michael, a senior, was studying to be an architect. We were introduced through mutual friends, and in two months' time we were dating exclusively.

Michael and I were typical college kids, full of hope and enthusiasm for the future. He had no trouble accepting my medical history, nor did any of my friends. Although I'd had cancer, I didn't see how it could present any obstacles to the plans I envisioned. If anything, beating the disease had made me more resilient and confident in my abilities.

The fall semester arrived, and with it came the realization that Michael would soon be graduating. He planned to move back to Pittsburgh and join his father's architectural firm, where he would be groomed to eventually take over. But Michael and I were very much in love; there was no way we could be apart. We talked about a future together, and then one day, ring in hand, he proposed.

As the chill of winter settled on Boulder, I began to make plans for the wedding and our life together. Michael and I decided that after the wedding we would move back East and I would finish school in Pennsylvania. But I was apprehensive. I'd never even been to Pittsburgh.

"That's easy enough to arrange," Michael said. "Why don't you come home with me for Thanksgiving? You can meet my parents and get to know the city."

And so I found myself in Pittsburgh on a cold and moonless November night. As Michael drove away from the airport, I confided how anxious I was. "Just relax and be yourself," he said with a smile. "The rest will work itself out."

Although it was late when we arrived, his parents were waiting up for us. We sat in the kitchen and chatted. Michael and I talked excitedly about our plans for the weekend and the neighborhoods of Pittsburgh we hoped to scout for houses. His parents said very little, and I thought it odd. I'd always known Michael to be open and affable, yet his parents seemed subdued, almost distant. But I was tired and more than a little nervous. So I dismissed those first impressions, sure that a good night's sleep would give me a fresh take on my prospective in-laws.

The following morning, Michael's mother agreed to join us for a tour of the city. When we stopped at a restaurant for lunch, she and I sat alone for a few minutes while Michael parked the car. We were trading polite "getting-to-know-you" small talk, when out of the blue she asked, "So what's it like living with a time bomb inside you?"

The question stunned me. Was she joking? A look into her expressionless face told me that this was no attempt at gallows humor. Unsure of what to say, I smiled nervously while shrugging my shoulders, and frantically glanced around the restaurant for a sign of my fiancé.

But Michael's arrival did little to disperse the tension between his mother and me. As soon as we returned to the house I told him what had happened. His reaction surprised me. Instead of becoming angry at his mother or empathizing with me, Michael responded with a dismissive shrug. "Oh, Susan," he said in his breezy manner, "you're being too sensitive. I'm sure she was just trying to make conversation."

Perhaps he was right. Although I was still upset, I was determined to overlook the incident.

That evening, Michael's father took us all out for dinner. Michael and his mother were engrossed in conversation when I turned to my future father-in-law and began to chat him up regarding our wedding plans.

"You know, Susan," he began slowly, "I'm sure you can understand my concern . . . as Michael's father . . ." He stared down at the food on his plate and nervously poked at it with his fork. "It's just that . . ." He seemed to want to say more, but was clearly having trouble finding the words to explain himself in detail. Instead, he simply cut to the chase. "It's just that . . . well, I don't want my son to be a widower."

In the abrupt and awkward silence that followed, I struggled with what to say. I was young and scared and completely intimidated by his attitude. I knew that if I tried to defend myself, I'd fall apart. Instead I let the remark pass, and, turning to my fiancé, quickly changed the subject.

Once Michael and I were alone, I recounted the remark made by his father. My fiancé brushed it aside with a wave of his hand. Although I assured him that this was no exaggeration, Michael felt that I was overplaying the incident. He could not, or would not, confront his parents. He continued to defend them, obliquely suggesting I be more grown-up about it. I told him I wasn't comfortable staying in their house and would prefer to spend the rest of the weekend in a nearby hotel. I went upstairs to pack, hoping he would join me.

But Michael remained downstairs with his parents. I finished packing my bags, slipped off my engagement ring, and placed it on the bedside table. Shattered and demoralized, I flew home the next day to Palo Alto, California, and my family.

At the time, Michael and his parents' behavior seemed incomprehensible and unforgivable. It wasn't until years later, when a mutual friend mentioned that Michael's uncle had died of cancer shortly before our engagement, that I began to understand the emotional subtext of that weekend in Pittsburgh. My fiancé had never mentioned his uncle's long illness, which had apparently taken a tremendous toll on the family. I now realized that Michael's parents wanted to protect their son from further pain, and in their eyes my medical history jeopardized his happiness. That in turn explained Michael's actions — or more precisely, his inaction. He was undoubtedly afraid that our marriage would anger his parents and was paralyzed by the choice he had to make.

In the months that followed, I did my best to forget about

Michael. I moved to San Francisco, where I took a job as a sales representative for a large cosmetics firm. It wasn't long before I formed a close friendship with Ellen, a young colleague who worked alongside me in the marketing department.

Our regional manager informed us that once we had completed our training we would be promoted and given our own territories to handle. I was looking forward to my promotion since I loved to travel. When a territory opened up in the Southwest, Ellen and I learned that the firm planned to cover it with someone from our office. The company was conducting interviews at its New York headquarters, so we both cleared our schedules for the trip.

"I've already booked a flight," Ellen announced when she dropped by my desk one morning. "I'm leaving the day after tomorrow. What about you?"

I couldn't leave until the following week. I wished her luck and told her not to be nervous.

I called Ellen the night she returned home, hoping to pick her brain about the interview. She sounded surprised to hear from me.

"So how did it go?" I asked.

She hesitated. "Well, I think I got the job."

"You mean they've already decided?"

"Yes. I guess they have."

I congratulated Ellen, but my enthusiasm was muted. Why hadn't I been given a chance to interview? The vice president of marketing had said he wanted to talk to both of us. What caused him to change his mind? I started asking questions and checking around. One day while having lunch with Kay, a company manager, I found the answer.

"I probably shouldn't even be telling you this," Kay began, "but it was such a lousy thing for them to do. I really thought you should know." She paused and leaned forward. "Ellen got the job because she told them you had cancer."

My mouth was dry, and I suddenly found it difficult to speak. I was as confused by Kay's revelation as I was shocked by Ellen's betrayal. My bout with cancer had been years before. The success of my treatment appeared total, my long-term prognosis a relative certainty. My doctors had even used the word "cured." I simply didn't understand. How could cancer still be a factor in my eligibility for promotion? Kay must have seen the bewilderment in my face.

"Ellen said that because you'd had cancer and it had affected your leg, you wouldn't be physically able to handle all the traveling the job required."

Like a blow on a bruise, her words revived the pain and anger I'd felt in Pittsburgh. How many years would have to pass before others saw me as a normal person? I knew that cancer was a chronic illness, but then, so was heart disease. And yet, I told Kay, coronaries weren't preventing many of the men we knew from getting ahead. Why should cancer be any different?

"The Big C scares most people," Kay observed. "They still think it's a death sentence, and they don't know how to deal with someone who's had it. If I were you, I'd keep my medical history under my hat. Save yourself the grief."

But Kay wasn't me, and she'd never faced a life-threatening illness. I'd fought hard to beat cancer, and I was fiercely proud of my victory. Yet I knew that Kay was right. There were others who viewed my experience as a taint rather than a triumph. During my recovery, I had made up my mind that I wasn't going to let the disease limit my goals and ambitions. But now, with a growing sense of outrage, I realized that cancer was continuing to reroute my life and cloud my future. I wanted it to stop.

I knew I had to leave the company. My self-esteem had been eroded, and I didn't have the fortitude to fight back. I'm not sure I would have known where to start.

I eventually found another job promoting a new line of cosmetics. But I was no fool. When people at work inquired about my treatment-induced limp, I told them it was the result of a skiing accident. I hated having to lie about something of which I was in no way ashamed, but I knew all too well that the truth could sabotage me. So I tucked that part of my life away, concealing it from others as if it were something sinister.

By my twenty-fifth birthday, I felt as though I'd firmly established myself and was fulfilled in both my personal and professional life. My cancer history continued to shadow me, however. The disease had created fissures in my life that I'd spent years trying to cover up, and I was beginning to understand how it had deeply affected my self-image. I knew cancer was a part of my identity, yet I felt tremendous pressure to deny that aspect of my life. I was strong, healthy, and ambitious. But was I really a "well" person if others saw me as less than healthy? And what if the cancer came back? Was I wasting my time planning for a future that might not happen?

It had taken me several years just to begin asking myself these questions, and as I sought answers the view I had of myself began to change.

To help reestablish myself, I moved down the coast to Los Angeles. I was no stranger to L.A.; I'd lived the first eighteen years of my life there. I enjoyed being back among old friends and familiar haunts. I landed a position as special events director for a large department store. The job was exciting, and I funneled most of my time and energy into it.

Despite my fresh start, I continued to feel strangely unsettled. I couldn't seem to shake a pervasive sense of frustration and anger, an accumulation of unresolved emotions that I knew had their genesis in my experience with cancer. The permanent damage caused by treatment fueled my anger. Cancer had altered my body image, and I had yet to accept and fully integrate those changes. My medical history had at various times undermined my employability, my insurability, even my social life. My old approach to dealing with the disease — to dodge and deny — didn't seem to be working anymore.

A sense of isolation compounded my anger. I hadn't found anyone in Los Angeles I could talk to about my problems as a survivor. I started seeing a psychotherapist, and that helped. But as understanding as she was, my therapist couldn't fully grasp the inner turmoil generated by my cancer experience. Friends were no different. "Hey, you survived," they would chide me. "You shouldn't be complaining. You're one of the lucky ones." I couldn't argue with their logic. But it didn't alleviate the feelings I had, and it certainly didn't diminish my anger.

A friend suggested I look for answers in a cancer support group. That made perfect sense to me. If I was going to find empathy anywhere, I would find it among people whose lives had also been touched by cancer. I attended one group, and another, then a third. However, these groups were composed of patients, people who were still fighting for their lives. My needs were different. I had won that fight. No one could fully appreciate how I was continuing to struggle with the ramifications of the disease.

No one, that is, except Lisa. She understood because she too was a survivor, though her battles were much more harrowing than mine.

I'd first met Lisa Jamison when I was eighteen, shortly after finishing cancer treatment at Stanford Medical Center. Once I had recovered enough to return to college, I arranged to drive back to Boulder with an acquaintance. On the way, my traveling companion suggested we stop in Lake Tahoe. She had a good friend living there whom she wanted me to meet, someone who had also recently completed cancer treatment.

Lisa and I hit it off immediately. She was my age and, like me, had undergone treatment at Stanford. Diagnosed at age fifteen with malignant teratoma, an ovarian cancer, Lisa underwent two years of aggressive therapy. Now she was in remission.

We spent hours comparing notes, talking about the doctors we both knew, and swapping war stories about our cancer treatments. We also shared a mordant sense of humor about our post-treatment complications. We'd joke about how, thanks to the effects of radiation treatment, we could now get a tan in two minutes. Lisa especially enjoyed describing how she used to rattle friends by telling them to turn off the lights so they could see her glow in the dark.

As I left Lake Tahoe, we agreed to stay in touch. And we did, running up exorbitant telephone bills in the process. Lisa and I shared all that was transferable of our cancer experience. We had both seen relationships change, career goals become distorted, health

insurance evaporate — all because of cancer. We worried about recurrence, our prospects for parenthood, and the long-term consequences of treatment.

For Lisa, those consequences were already formidable. Her cancer had been particularly virulent, and in a last-ditch effort to turn
the tide, she had received extremely high doses of radiation. In her
case, however, it had been too much of a good thing; the radiotherapy had caused severe adhesions in her abdomen. Adhesions also
affected the arteries in her legs, progressively diminishing her ability
to walk. Although she had numerous operations to repair the damage, nothing seemed to offer long-term relief.

"I think my radiologist has a crush on me," Lisa would joke from
her hospital bed. "Why else would he have rigged it so I have to
come back here all the time?" Lisa had a marvelous gift for disguis-
ing adversity, but sometimes the painful ordeals would overwhelm
her. "If this is the cure, give me back the disease," she once remarked, her voice cracking with bitterness. But those moments were
few and far between. Even during her darkest times, Lisa's irrepressible optimism would eventually burst through the gloom.

But I was alarmed. Why hadn't Lisa been warned that these
complications might arise? What sort of long-term effects of treatment might *I* expect in the future? The need for answers consumed
me. I scoured libraries for books, articles, reports, anything that
would shed light on our concerns as survivors. Nothing came close
to providing adequate information. Every book I read on cancer
dealt with the immediate needs of patients fighting the disease, de-
tailing modes of treatment, emotional coping, and the issues of
death and dying. But what about people who were living *after* cancer? Scores of books existed on the lifestyle problems faced by cardiac patients, diabetics, and alcoholics. Why weren't there similar
books providing practical, long-term support for cancer survivors? I
told Lisa about my futile search for information. "It's as if we'd been
dropped in the middle of a desert," she observed, "and left to fend
for ourselves."

By 1985 Lisa's health had further deteriorated and she was back in the hospital, this time to undergo a colostomy. I felt helpless watching her struggle to recuperate from yet another operation, but I did what I could to cheer her up. "When you're back on your feet," I told her, "let's plan a vacation together. Somewhere sunny and warm, where we can kick back and relax."

Two months later, Lisa called me from San Francisco. "Palm Springs," she announced. "You suggested we take a trip together, and I'm ready to go. Next weekend, okay?"

It was the perfect prescription. The hot dry weather lifted Lisa's spirits and seemed to help her feel better physically. On our first day in Palm Springs, we talked long into the night about our lives and hopes for the future. As always, our conversation inevitably circled back to the subject of surviving cancer. As we talked, we vented our frustration. Why wasn't anyone addressing these issues?

Lisa reminded me. "Susan, you have to remember that the medical community is focused mainly on treating the disease, not what comes after the cure." Between sips of iced tea she added, "If we want answers, we may have to provide them ourselves, or at least start the discussion. I think it's time we stop complaining and start doing."

I knew she was right. If we couldn't find a support group for survivors, why not create one ourselves? On the spot, Lisa and I decided to join forces and do just that. We began brainstorming, imagining an organization that would provide its members with peer support groups, professional counseling, and educational programs.

We continued our brainstorming session the next day. Lisa sat in the hot desert sun, all but hidden under a big floppy hat, a yellow legal pad propped on her knees. On her notepad she outlined goals and jotted down objectives, giving shape and structure to our ideas. Many hours and legal pads later, Lisa abruptly looked up at me and said, "Cancervive. Let's call it Cancervive."

By the end of that weekend we had laid the groundwork for our new organization. We drove back to Los Angeles, and Lisa flew on to San Francisco. We were feeling exhilarated and hopeful, eager to get started on making our weekend dream a reality.

Then tragedy struck. On her return home, Lisa's complications flared up and she was forced to reenter the hospital. The massive dose of radiation she'd received was now causing the major arteries in her pelvis and legs to close off. First a foot had to be amputated, then her entire leg. Several months later, doctors removed the other leg. I flew up to San Francisco, devastated by what had happened to my friend. I was also terrified. How could I be sure that what was happening to Lisa wouldn't one day happen to me?

Lisa saw the fear in my eyes. "Don't worry, Susan, you're going to be okay. After all, I'm counting on you to get Cancervive going." Then she smiled. "Just promise me you'll hold on to that leg of yours, all right?"

Lisa's ferocious fighting spirit gave me the inspiration I needed. I returned to Los Angeles and immediately started organizing the paperwork and getting the word out about a newly chartered non-profit organization called Cancervive. I contacted newspapers, magazines, television stations, and hospitals. I was sure that hundreds, perhaps thousands, of survivors were encountering problems similar to those Lisa and I had faced. It was just a matter of reaching them.

A few weeks later I was asked to appear on a national television talk show. The simple act of telling my story had an amazingly cathartic effect, not only on me, it seemed, but on other survivors who saw it. After my appearance the station was swamped with calls from survivors who had telephoned to say, in essence, "That's me. That's my life. Just change the name."

Lisa and I were elated by the response. We knew then that our reasons for starting Cancervive were valid.

I decided to keep the first support group meeting small and informal so that those attending would feel comfortable about speaking their minds. The group that gathered in my living room on a warm July evening in 1985 included two oncology social workers; Nadia, an eight-year survivor of Hodgkin's disease; and Jon, a young man who had finished treatment for a brain tumor six months before and was now in remission. I had no agenda planned. Instead, I suggested that we talk about our experiences as survivors, raising any and all issues that concerned us.

At first it was hard for Jon and Nadia to talk about themselves. Jon explained why.

"I'm uncomfortable talking about the negative aspects of surviving," he said. "I certainly don't want to sound like some kind of ingrate."

"That's okay," I responded. "Then if you don't mind, I'll start." I talked about my life, my bout with cancer, and the problems I encountered once I'd left the hospital. It wasn't easy speaking to a group of strangers, confiding some of my deepest fears and relating the pain and anger I'd kept bottled up inside for ten years. And yet, even though I hardly knew these people, I felt they weren't really strangers. They seemed to understand what I was saying and how I was feeling in a way only a survivor could.

"I don't think I'm alone," I said in conclusion. "I think these issues affect all survivors in one way or another, regardless of age or prognosis. I'm worried that other people will go through what I went through, and that they may take too long, as I did, to come to terms with the legacy of their cancer."

The room was silent for a few moments. Then Nadia spoke. "My boyfriend and I have talked about maybe getting married in a year or two, and it's made me think a lot about whether or not I can have children. I recently asked my doctor about it. He said that treatment may have left me infertile; he'd have to do some tests to be sure. It took a while for that news to sink in, but once it did, I cried for days. Now I'm wondering, how do I tell my boyfriend? I'm so worried that it will change everything."

Jon nodded and said, "Now that I'm in remission, I can't stop thinking about a recurrence. With my kind of cancer, there's a good chance of that happening. My doctor says I shouldn't worry about it, that I should just put it out of my mind and get on with my life. But he isn't offering me any guarantees of a cure either. At least when I was getting radiation, I felt I had some protection. Being off treatment scares the hell out of me. I keep waiting for the other shoe to drop. How am I supposed to deal with that?"

I knew there were no easy answers to Jon's question, or Nadia's, or mine. But as we talked, a bond began to form among the members of this tiny nucleus of a support group. The more open we were about what had happened to us, the more unburdened we felt. I could empathize with Nadia's dilemma because it was my concern as well. I knew Jon's fear because I had faced it too. Our lives touched and crossed at a juncture called cancer, and it was there that we recognized ourselves in each other.

This was the beginning of Cancervive, the organization Lisa and I hoped would represent the needs and concerns of all survivors. The problems that Jon, Nadia, Lisa, and I faced weren't unique; they were just a few of the challenges that form the backdrop to life after cancer.

2
Making the Transition to the Well World

I celebrated my twenty-first birthday as a cancer patient at the University of Texas M. D. Anderson Cancer Center in Houston. My parents threw a party for me in the hospital, and we asked everyone on my floor to attend. But we were celebrating more than just my birthday. The day before, my oncologist had presented me with the best present of all: he told me I was in remission.

I couldn't wait to get home, gain back my strength, and get on with my life. But a funny thing happened on my way back to the well world. Several weeks after leaving the hospital, I couldn't seem to shake a growing sense of anxiety. The care and support I'd received during my hospital stay had provided me with a sense of security. But now, on my own, I felt abandoned, disoriented, frightened. I wasn't sure how to fit back into the outside world anymore.

— Anita, three-year survivor of osteosarcoma

REMISSION. No other word is as liberating and exhilarating to the cancer patient. Remission means an end to the grueling round of treatments and tests, of countless visits with your medical team. It signals a return to health and, for most, the eventual reappearance of hair and vitality. In short, remission means gaining back a sense of normality and getting on with life.

Or does it? Although this transitional period is outwardly a happy, celebratory one, survivors frequently find their joy tempered by unanticipated problems and unexpected emotions. When Anita shared her story with a Cancervive support group, we could immediately identify with her experience. Like Anita, many survivors leave the hospital with ambivalence, frightened and overwhelmed by the seemingly formidable idea of making the transition back to "normal" everyday life. They soon discover, as I did, that safe passage back to the well world isn't as easy as simply walking out the oncologist's door. Because cancer is a chronic disease, and therefore one that requires lifelong monitoring, it takes time to adjust to a new sense of normalcy.

The road to recovery can be pitted with potholes, and some survivors wonder why they never received much in the way of advance warnings. One reason is that the psychosocial education of the recovered cancer patient is a relatively new field. Health care professionals now know that the post-treatment hardships that cancer patients have to endure are not only physical in nature. With the dramatic rise of survival rates and long-term remission in recent years, it has become increasingly apparent that the psychological and social consequences of the disease are just as important as those that are physical in nature.

Dr. Michael B. Van Scoy-Mosher, an oncologist at Cedars-Sinai Medical Center in Los Angeles, is one of the growing number of doctors who concur with this view. "A lot of physicians feel that once cancer treatment is complete, the patient's problems are over and life goes on," says Dr. Van Scoy-Mosher. "But some of the greatest problems I've seen actually *begin* then. From my standpoint, the survivorship phase is one of the most challenging and in many ways the most difficult periods in the cancer patient's life."

Dr. Van Scoy-Mosher adds that the immediate post-treatment phase is a particularly vulnerable time. For instance, it is not uncommon for recovering patients to feel enormous anxiety about going off treatment or parting ways with the hospital staff. Many survivors have difficulty regaining a sense of control and direction in their lives, whereas others struggle with depression, fatigue, or delayed stress reactions to their cancer experience. Through this process of "normalization," the questions and concerns never stop percolating: "What happens now? How will I fit back in? How can I be sure the cancer is gone?" In this chapter, you will meet several survivors who wrestled with these questions as they made their break from the acute stage of cancer care.

Breaking Free of the Hospital World

When Robert, a college student now in his fourth year of remission, first came to our support group, he struck me as a very self-assured, confident young man. He described how during his year and a half of chemotherapy for Hodgkin's disease, his sights were set on the day he would be free from the world of needles, nurses, and nausea. But as Robert explained, when that time came he discovered that his relief was mingled with other, unexpected emotions.

ℰ I'd always considered myself pretty much of an "in-control" guy, and I'd never had a problem with separation anxiety before. But then again, I'd never had cancer. And I'd never been stuck in a hospital for so long.

It's ironic, because I'd always had a phobia of hospitals. I hated the idea of even visiting them. And then — *boom* — there I was, forced to be a patient. I couldn't wait to be rid of the place, all the bland food and round-the-clock tests.

As I approached the end of my treatment protocol, I was naturally relieved to be getting away from all that. But to my surprise, I was also upset by it. I wasn't so worried about the cancer anymore; in fact, my oncologist even wrote a guarantee on my insurance form stating that I wouldn't get a recurrence. What I did feel was strong separation anxiety as the medical team slowly started to withdraw their attention. I suddenly realized how emotionally dependent I'd become on the hospital staff, even the chemo. I tried talking to my oncologist about it but his attitude seemed to be, "Hey, I have lots of sick people to treat."

I know it sounds crazy, and I'm more than a little embarrassed even admitting it, but I felt as though I'd been discarded. I was angry about it and anxious, even panicky at times. I could handle those feelings during the day, but the nights could be tough. &b

Robert certainly isn't the only survivor who worries about parting ways with the oncology ward. Anita, the survivor you met at the beginning of this chapter, expressed a similar concern. To someone who has never experienced a serious disease, anxiety over leaving the hospital might seem odd or overblown. But even those who receive outpatient treatment can become psychologically dependent on the medical world. Many survivors readjust fairly easily to normal life, but others may be plagued for weeks or months by mood swings, low self-esteem, and an undercurrent of anxiety.

When you think about it, those feelings are quite normal, even predictable. After all, a cancer diagnosis transforms your life. It also transfers some of the responsibility for your well-being to a group of relative strangers. Over time, however, these health care professionals may become like a second family. With your cancer diagnosis as the call to arms, they united with you in the fight for your life. They saw you at your worst, and they were there to cheer your victories. So it should come as no surprise that you have, perhaps unconsciously, developed strong psychological bonds with them.

Julie Steckel, a licensed clinical social worker in Los Angeles who works with recovering cancer patients, finds that it's common for survivors to feel ambivalent about leaving the hospital world.

&b Quite a bit of psychological retooling takes place once cancer patients leave the acute phase of treatment. For some, it's difficult to let go of the sick role and all of the dependency and attention that goes with it. Many survivors are worried about leaving the safe, secure hospital environment. They may feel they are being abandoned at an extremely precarious time by some of the very people who have been most concerned for their well-being. Often this concern is compounded by the fear of recurrence, which is usually most intense at this time.

Then again, many survivors have the problem of readjusting to their previous lifestyles. They are no longer caught up in the intense drama that a crisis like cancer represents, and so they need to shift their focus to normal everyday activities. All these changes can result in anxiety, fear, depression, and anger. ॐ

Leaving Treatment Behind

As unpleasant as cancer therapy can be, many survivors dread the day it ends. When the oncologist announces the end of treatment, a patient's first reaction may be one of anxiety. "How will I live without it?"

That's the question Cory keeps asking herself. The fifty-six-year-old neonatal nurse was diagnosed with breast cancer three years ago. A biopsy following her mastectomy revealed that the disease had affected eleven lymph nodes. It had invaded Cory's chest wall and metastasized to her liver and spine.

But after prolonged treatment, Cory's physicians told her that the long, intensive course of chemotherapy and radiation had worked; her cancer was in remission. She found to her surprise that she felt ambivalent:

ॐ I've been on chemotherapy for three years now. Other than barfing up my insides all the time, I think I handled it pretty well. Now my oncologist tells me that I can quit chemo soon. He thinks it's great news, and I do too, except that I'm also scared to death. Chemo has been my security blanket. After all, it's a rare instance when a patient experiences a recurrence while receiving chemotherapy.

This isn't the first time I've faced this fear. After my second year of treatment, I was told I could probably go off it soon. Then my doctors took another look at my tests and decided that, just to be sure, I should get another year of chemo. I heard that and all I could think was, Oh, good! I don't have to worry about dying for another year. Chemo has almost become a way of life for me. I feel like an addict. Next month is my last month of treatment. I don't know how I'm going to handle it, knowing that I won't have those chemicals blasting away at any stray cancer cells. &ob;

Robert experienced a similar problem when he ended his treatment for Hodgkin's disease.

&ob; I first started noticing what I call my "withdrawal symptoms," right after my last chemotherapy treatment. When it came time to quit, it was just like going cold turkey. I really believed the treatment was all that was keeping me alive. I guess that's what was so psychologically addicting about it. It took me a while to realize that I had been just as important in the fight against my cancer as those drugs. &ob;

Recovering patients frequently use expressions like "cold turkey" and "withdrawal symptoms" when describing the psychological rigors of going off treatment. Some patients actually request that their treatment be prolonged, even though there is no medical reason for doing so.

As anxiety-provoking as the termination of treatment can be, it's important to remember that too much medicine is as bad as too little. "Patients need to realize that everything we are currently using to treat cancer comes with its own set of problems," asserts Dr. Richard J. Steckel, chairman of the Radiological Sciences Department at UCLA's School of Medicine.

&ob; The aim of oncology today is to balance any harmful side effects with the goal of getting the patient into remission. Surgery, radiation, and chemotherapy often serve only as a means of pushing the balance of that fight in favor of the body. When all is said and done, it is the patient's own body that ultimately wields control over cancer. &ob;

However, termination of treatment signals an end to the reassuring routine of hospital surveillance. During treatment, you may have felt as if your lifeline was hooked to that antiseptic world, and so the hospital became a haven offering womblike security. But no one can stay in the womb forever. Sooner or later, you have to start living the life cancer forced you to put on hold.

How do you emotionally disengage yourself from the hospital world? Several Cancervive members have succeeded by simply easing themselves back into everyday activities. You might try to do this by quickly reestablishing old patterns and routines in your work, school, or family life. Focus on activities you enjoy or find worthwhile, and at a pace you can handle, so that you can feel as if you are reinvesting yourself in the well world. Another way to allay anxiety is to protect your newfound health through a change in lifestyle habits. This is the approach Cory chose:

& I realized I could freak out over my withdrawal from chemotherapy, or I could take an active part in building myself up and bolstering my immune system. During the last year or two I've become very interested in how diet, nutrition, and stress seem to influence the body's immune response to diseases. I read somewhere that more than seventy percent of cancers are due to lifestyle habits. So I've made a concerted effort to change a lot of my old habits. No more high-fat foods, no more couch potato routine. I'm even learning how to meditate. I guess you could say I've adopted a holistic approach to the way I'm going to live my life. My kids think it's fantastic. I'll admit it isn't always easy — I still sneak an occasional ice cream cone — but it is giving me a new sense of being in charge of my health. It also gives me peace of mind to know that I'm doing the best I can. The rest I'm just going to have to leave to the man upstairs. &

Anita found that her anxieties were best addressed in group therapy. She says that the feedback, support, and comradeship of other survivors kept her from falling into a state of helplessness. It also provided her with a few tips on how to handle her fears.

& The first step for me was to face up to my feelings. By talking to other survivors, I discovered that I wasn't the only person who felt scared and disoriented after being released from the hospital. I was so relieved to know that it was okay to have those feelings. One of the people in my group said that the way she took care of her "remission blues" was to do hospital volunteer work once a week. Those weekly visits to familiar surroundings somehow reassure her and allow her to feel as if she's in control of the situation. I think I might try doing that. &

Robert's approach to post-treatment anxiety was through yet another route.

& I decided to drop in on one of the social workers I'd come to know during treatment. I talked to her about the difficulty I was having psychologically weaning myself from chemotherapy and hospital care. She suggested that, because my oncologist wasn't very receptive to my problem, I talk to one of the other doctors on my treatment team. Ultimately I did connect with another oncologist, a colleague of the doctor who treated me. Although this oncologist had not been involved in my treatment, he knew my case and all the details. But more important, he was very receptive to my concerns. He said my anxiety was normal and that in time it would diminish and disappear. We talked about the specifics of my follow-up schedule and the particular symptoms I should watch for. In the meantime, he suggested I call him whenever I needed to talk, or as he put it, "plug in." His advice helped a lot. Now the time between my three-month checkups doesn't seem like an eternity. And what's more, I'm back to getting a good night's sleep. &

One of these methods may work for you, but they are certainly not the only means available. You may find, as I did, that the simple act of talking about your anxieties with someone else can lift your spirits. A survivor support group like Cancervive offers a forum in which these concerns can be addressed and coping techniques shared. If you're not comfortable in a group, find a friend or relative willing to lend an ear. But if you are having a difficult time readjusting after treatment and your anxiety is acute or prolonged, don't hesitate to seek professional help.

Renegotiating the Patient-Doctor Relationship

> Tell me and I will forget.
> Show me and I will remember.
> Involve me and I will understand.
> — Chinese proverb

It's natural for recovered cancer patients to feel emotionally tied to the hospital when it has provided them with the medicine and machinery for successfully treating their disease. But occasionally survivors find themselves struggling with a more personal kind of bond: the traditional patient-doctor relationship.

Physicians have long held a revered place in society. Many of us were brought up to believe that doctors can do no wrong — that they are beyond reproach, even beyond questioning. When we're sick, we depend on them to marshal the forces of modern medicine on our behalf. Who are we to doubt them?

Although this traditional, paternalistic view still exists, it is changing. Roles are being redefined because of the rise of patient advocates and the Patients Bill of Rights, endorsed in 1992 by the American Hospital Association. In addition, health care management has undergone a profound shift in recent decades, with health maintenance programs putting a considerable strain on the patient-doctor relationship.

Most of us are now aware of how essential it is to approach medical care as informed and responsible "consumers." Through access to the Internet, we now have at our fingertips access to a vast bank of clinical medical advice and information, and it has helped to transform the consumer-provider relationship. After all, knowledge is power; why shouldn't shared knowledge translate into shared power?

If you consider it odd to view yourself as a health care consumer and your doctor a "provider," you may want to ask yourself why. After all, oncology is a business — a big business. Without you and consumers like you, the machinery of this multibillion-dollar industry would grind to a halt. As an empowered patient, you have every right to ask questions, expect answers you can understand, and make health care decisions accordingly.

According to Cedars-Sinai's Dr. Van Scoy-Mosher, there are two extreme versions of the patient-doctor relationship.

&% At one end of the spectrum is the paternalistic approach, where the doctor is the authority figure. He makes all the decisions as to what the patient needs. The other extreme is that of consumer sovereignty, where the doctor hands the patient a laundry list of possible choices and then lets the patient decide. Somewhere in between these two approaches is a relationship based on shared decision-making. &%

As the consumer, it is your responsibility to be as medically literate as possible about your type of cancer as well as what you as a survivor can do to stay healthy. Learn how to listen effectively and try to be both reasonable and realistic in what you can expect from your health care provider. Doctors, on the other hand, have the responsibility of understanding the consumer's fears and concerns and imparting their medical advice in language that is clear and concise. To get the most out of this relationship, you should strive to become partners with your primary care physician. As with any partnership, you should both have equal say in the decision-making process. As in all relationships, honesty, trust, and communication are essential to making it work.

Effective communication and mutual respect can help you to better understand and comply with your physician's recommendations and provide you with increased confidence, bolster your assertiveness, and give you greater control over the quality of care you receive.

Dr. Van Scoy-Mosher adds, "Both health care provider and consumer, on either end of the stethoscope, should listen to and develop empathy for the other."

But there are times when either the doctor isn't listening or the patient isn't communicating, and as a result, empathy is in short supply. Five years ago, a forty-nine-year-old Cancervive member named Dana underwent a modified double mastectomy. While she was recuperating, her surgeon told her that because there was no lymph node involvement, she wouldn't require any further treatment. But Dana's elation over the news was soon undercut by the anger she felt toward her doctor.

ॐ I went into the mastectomy operation counting on the surgeon to save my life. At that point, I trusted him implicitly. I thought he was like God, this omnipotent authority figure. And, of course, I was the typical passive patient.

After my surgery, just before I left the hospital, I asked my doctor what I needed to do from that point on. What should I watch out for? Was there anything I could do to control the swelling in my left arm? He answered rather brusquely. "No, not really. Just be sure to get a chest x-ray every year." With that, he turned and left the room. I was completely stunned by his cavalier attitude. He had just removed both my breasts, and he was treating me as if I'd had a mole removed. He could see that I was upset and scared. He knew I needed answers to questions. Instead he acted like a jerk. His interest was in the disease, not me, the patient. I felt as if I had been summarily booted out the door. Were all my follow-up visits with him going to be like this? ॐ

Unfortunately, not all patient-doctor relationships run smoothly, no matter how much energy or trust you invest. Left unresolved, both Dana's anger and her doctor's attitude posed a threat to her compliance with follow-up care. Ultimately, there is only one question Dana, as well as virtually all survivors, need to ask themselves: Is the relationship I have with my doctor good for my health? If you can't answer with a resounding yes, consider switching to another primary-care physician.

Of course, if you've diagnosed a problem in the relationship, you should attempt to speak frankly about it with your doctor. Doing so may spark a solution. Then again, it may not. But at least you'll know you tried. There are any number of reasons why you might need to make a switch. For instance, changing health care plans may require you to find another doctor if your current physician isn't enrolled in your new plan. What you do will ultimately hinge on your particular circumstances and needs. Should you have trouble reaching a decision, consider speaking to a health care advocate (also known as patient representatives), whose job it is to act as a liaison between hospital staff and patients. Health care advocates can be excellent allies when it comes to mediating between doctors and patients.

Dana told me that it was the anger she felt over her doctor's attitude that prompted her to attend a Cancervive support group. Dana is no wallflower, and she used her first group meeting to vent her rage. She talked with other survivors and compared notes on their patient-doctor relationships.

⇌ I listened to a couple of other women describe their mastectomy experiences, and I suddenly felt like I had gone through mine with blinders on. They helped me see that although my mastectomy was performed by a competent surgeon, he also happened to be an insensitive and uncommunicative doctor. I slowly came to understand that he was, after all, only human. That diffused a lot of my anger and really opened my eyes to the kind of patient I had been. Now I'm no longer passive when it comes to my own well-being. I made the decision not to go back to this doctor for follow-ups. Since then, I've found a physician who has a terrific bedside manner. He really takes the time to listen and was tremendously helpful in guiding me to another surgeon for breast reconstruction. I'm finally beginning to appreciate how my cancer experience changed me; it made me more alert to my health, more self-reliant and assertive as a patient. And that in turn has affected my relationship with doctors. &⁊

The termination of therapy can be an especially vulnerable time in the patient-doctor relationship. As the patient approaches the end of treatment, visits to the doctor's office take less and less time, until that last appointment. This meeting can be so short and cursory that many people end up feeling as if they have been somehow deserted, left alone to deal with the uncertainties of recovery. Says social worker Julie Steckel:

&⁊ Many times the doctor tells the patient in essence, "I've done my part in this joint victory; you won't be needing me as much anymore." This is often the doctor's way of letting go. However, because the patient is dependent on the doctor, he or she may experience the break as a personal abandonment, even a betrayal. The end of treatment is really the end of an era, so to speak, and one that needs to be acknowledged by both the patient and the doctor. &⁊

Few physicians learn how to handle the emotional dynamics that accompany the end of the patient-doctor relationship. This is not to imply that all physicians are insensitive to the emotional concerns of their patients; many are very supportive. Nonetheless, the majority of physicians still believe that a patient's psychosocial problems are more appropriately the domain of social workers and other therapists. Also, because of the considerable demands of their work schedules, increasingly burdened in recent times by the constraints of managed care, physicians frequently remain detached from the people they treat in order not to become overwhelmed, both emotionally and professionally. But all too often, patients interpret such behavior as defensive, unresponsive, or uncaring.

I don't mean to suggest that the doctor is always to blame when problems arise between patient and physician. Like Dana, many of us are rather passive when addressing members of the medical community. As a health care consumer, however, you have duties and responsibilities. Don't forget that *you* are an integral part of the health care team; your input is essential. When lines of communication between patient and doctor aren't as open as they should be, both parties tend to second-guess each other, and misunderstandings can mushroom into crises. Of course, there will always be those individuals for whom ignorance is bliss. Some people simply cope better with few facts and plenty of faith. This is a perfectly acceptable approach, provided it works for and not against you.

Dr. Richard Steckel, chairman of the Radiological Department at UCLA's School of Medicine, believes that physicians and their patients should conduct a sort of "debriefing" session at the end of treatment.

& In many ways, it's just as important to leave the acute phase of treatment with the same kind of interview and review that the patient and doctor had at the time of the initial diagnosis or before treatment. It is particularly important for the patient to get as much information as he or she needs to ensure a successful recovery. Also, having this kind of information allows patients to establish a greater sense of control over their lives. &

The relationship between you and your doctor is unique. Its success will depend on a variety of factors, including both your personalities and your philosophical approaches to health care. And because cancer is a chronic disease, the relationship will continue long after treatment ends. This is why it's important to know you have the full support and cooperation of your physician.

The consumer-provider relationship is a two-way street. Be considerate of your doctor's tight schedule and challenging workload, and try not to be unrealistic in your expectations. As much as we might like to believe that doctors have all the answers, the reality is that they don't. If, like Dana, we insist on putting physicians on pedestals, we are bound to lose sight of them as human beings. Doctors aren't mind readers, and they aren't infallible. When something is bothering you, it's up to you to say so. As simplistic as that sounds, many of us have trouble remembering it.

If you find that the relationship with your doctor is becoming contaminated by anger or frustration, arrange to discuss the matter candidly, either directly with your physician or with one of his or her colleagues (such as the doctor who initially referred you). If you are unable to resolve your conflict, don't think twice about finding another physician who is more responsive to your needs.

Emotional Entanglements

Oncology wards are hardly anyone's idea of a place for romantic rendezvous. Nonetheless, some patients find themselves caught up in sexual fantasies involving one or more of the people on their medical team. (This is especially true of breast cancer patients because of the strong sexual identification of the female breast.) For most patients these feelings amount to nothing more than a harmless crush, but for others they can take a more ardent form. In either case, an emotional involvement can make breaking away from the hospital environment all the more difficult.

Monique, a fifty-two-year-old psychotherapist, underwent a mastectomy six years ago. Three years later she was operated on for stomach cancer, a malignancy unrelated to her previous breast cancer. She had surgery to remove her stomach and spleen and was given an intensive schedule of chemotherapy and radiation. Her prognosis was poor; the doctors gave her a 5 percent chance of survival. But Monique wasn't buying into the bleak statistics. Today she is in remission and back at work in her private practice.

艹 I didn't feel any of that anxiousness about going off treatment, like so many other survivors do. Instead, my problem was letting go of the relationship with my doctor.

When I first met the oncologist after my diagnosis for stomach cancer, he asked if there was anything he could do. I told him, "Yes! Don't look so damn sad when you talk to me!" I knew my prognosis wasn't great, but I didn't want to get a mindset. We ended up having a wonderful working relationship. He was very professional and understanding, and we did a lot of joking around as well. He never quoted me statistics, and he was never pessimistic or patronizing. He knew I was a psychotherapist and so he treated me like a colleague.

Several months into treatment I started fantasizing about him. When I did, I'd get very emotional about our relationship. Deep down, I knew I had to stop this crazy obsessing, but I just couldn't let go of it. Sometimes when I'd see him, reality would kick in. I'd realize how we both had happy, stable marriages, and that all this fantasizing was crazy. But then a few days later I'd find myself daydreaming about him all over again.

Once during an office visit he told me, rather offhandedly, that I was *one* of his favorite patients. I remember hearing that and then suddenly blurting out, "But I thought I was your *favorite!*" I couldn't believe the way I was behaving. I'd reacted just like a child. Fortunately, he was very diplomatic. He undoubtedly could sense what was going on with me.

The last time I saw him for treatment he said, "Good news! You won't have to see me for another three months." Now usually that's the kind of news every patient wants to hear. But not me. I remember thinking, Oh my God. What do I do now? After that, I would spend hours dreaming up reasons to call him just to have an excuse to chat. &%

Many women — and more than a few men — find that relations with their doctors become entangled in a web of seemingly crazy and confusing emotions. The dynamics of the traditional patient-doctor relationship can lay the groundwork for this. Some patients gain comfort and reassurance from a paternalistic approach in which the doctor acts as an authority figure and the patient dutifully follows orders. But because of the intense emotions that accompany a diagnosis of cancer, the patient's respect for the doctor can develop into more intimate feelings.

Patients may also project romantic feelings onto doctors as a sort of coping mechanism. Fantasizing can be an excellent way of deflecting or blotting out fear and anxiety. And why not? As survivors like Monique admit, daydreaming about the doctor is certainly a lot more pleasant than worrying about all the "what ifs" of cancer. Social worker Julie Steckel points out that this is one reason why the separation phase of the patient-doctor relationship can be particularly difficult for some women.

❧ Women have a tendency to make more emotional connections in their relationships, and they don't like having them broken. Men, on the other hand, often use separation as a way of delineating and setting boundaries in relationships. If the doctor is a man, an abrupt separation with the patient may be the only way he knows how to say goodbye.

It's quite normal to have romantic fantasies about a doctor. It's a function of our dependency needs in a time of crisis. Our first love is for our patients, and that kind of relationship is often duplicated in the patient-doctor relationship. Also, many women have romantic notions that are based in part on their fantasies of having a strong, protective lover, and that again ties in directly to aspects of the patient-doctor relationship. ❧

Of course, it can happen that a physician or a patient will attempt to take advantage of latent sexual fantasies or sexual attraction and act on them. That, of course, is a mistake. Any sexual relationship between a patient and a doctor, for whatever the reason, is a serious matter and constitutes a breach of professional boundaries. Such boundaries are there primarily for your protection — to set physical and emotional limits in order to maintain trust and respect. When such boundaries are crossed, it is usually the patient who is most negatively affected.

In the end, Monique's training as a psychotherapist helped her analyze her feelings and, in turn, understand what motivated them.

&b I was able to rationalize what I was doing and keep it in perspective. I realized that in this relationship the doctor was more important to me than I was to him. I was putting my life into his hands in the fervent hope that he would save it. He had become my knight in a white coat. After I figured that out, I started asking myself what it was that was missing in my life, what I was getting out of this infatuation. I would essentially do a therapy number on myself and that would keep my emotions in check. &b

These insights allowed Monique to see how emotionally dependent she had become on her physician. But sometimes the dynamics are reversed. Linda's relationship with her oncologist is an example. A forty-two-year-old computer consultant, Linda was eight years into remission on her initial diagnosis of leukemia when she began suffering from chronic flulike symptoms. She called her family doctor, who suggested she call her oncologist.

&b I had kept the same oncologist since my first diagnosis. He'd followed my progress, and I'd made a point of staying in touch with him. We had a very amicable relationship throughout my illness and recovery, but now that I look back on it I realize that perhaps the relationship was too close. In a way I had become like a trophy to him. I was one of his success stories; I was a *survivor.*

When I told him I wasn't feeling so great he refused to believe it might have anything to do with a recurrence. I finally insisted that he examine me for a possible malignancy. The tests came back positive — I had cancer again. He was devastated, and I wasn't too happy about it either. I had clearly not made his day.

My respect for him really took a nose dive after that. I felt used. My best interests were obviously not in the forefront of his mind. I was mad as hell, and very confused as to what to do. He's a skilled physician, a well-respected oncologist. I wanted him to treat me for this recurrence. But I sure didn't want to be just another feather in his cap. ஃ

When doctors let their own emotions get in the way, patients like Linda understandably feel angry and helpless. But Linda wanted to maintain the relationship with her doctor. She knew, however, that before she could reenter treatment under his care she had to clear the air.

ஃ I didn't want things to be poisoned by these bad vibes between us. I felt I'd get too emotional if I had a face-to-face talk with him, so I wrote him a letter instead. I told him that I could sense his disappointment in me for getting a recurrence. I asked him to put himself in my shoes. How did he think *I* felt? I explained that I needed a doctor who would continue to be optimistic and encouraging even if things weren't looking great. I asked him pointblank: "Can you provide me with that, along with the chemo?" If not, I said, I would find an oncologist who would.

He called me a few days later. He sounded pained by what had happened and apologized. He said, "I was upset that you of all people should have a relapse. I've known you a long time, and damn it, the news really shook me up." He said he hoped I would forgive him and added, "I hope you'll give me another chance. I feel confident that together we can beat it." I hung up the phone and felt so relieved that I cried. That telephone call did more for me than any medicine could. ஃ

Through the simple act of writing a letter, Linda renegotiated her patient-doctor relationship. Although she is facing another round with cancer, she tells me she still feels like a winner.

Checking the Facts with Your Health Care Team

In making your break from the hospital environment, you're bound to feel apprehensive about what lies ahead. This is the time to begin transitioning from the role of patient to that of survivor — a person with a history of cancer. It is extremely important to now shift your focus to the need for follow-up care. Certainly, the farther out from treatment you are, the more likely the disease will take a permanent back seat in your life. But keep in mind that primary responsibility for your health remains with you. Your cancer and its treatment may have resulted in physical and emotional changes that could take some time to understand. Some of these changes may be permanent or not yet evident. As you pass the acute stage of cancer care, arrange a time with your health care team. Take Dr. Steckel's advice and schedule a debriefing session. This can give you a sense of closure and provide direction for your future well-being. The following is a checklist of suggestions to guide you through your session.

- *Organize your meeting.* Before you schedule an appointment with your health care team, draw up a list of questions you want to ask. Use the most out of this time by prioritizing the questions you have concerning your health care needs. Knowledge is power, and it can greatly maximize your feelings of control and help maintain assertiveness. If you wish, bring a friend or relative to the meeting. Having a friend or family member in attendance may help to bolster you psychologically. Also, take along a tape-recorder. Doing so can reduce the chances that you will misinterpret or forget important information.

- *Learn the specifics on your diagnosis, treatment, prognosis, and possible post-treatment complications.* Be sure to get a copy of your medical records. This may require a written request, but it's well worth the effort involved. As years go by, you may lose track of important information concerning your case history. For instance, it may not seem very relevant to you to differentiate between stage 1 and stage 3 Hodgkin's disease, but it makes a tremendous difference to a physician. Ask about what you can do to alleviate any lingering side effects of treatment, and what you should look for in the way of any late or long-term effects. Learn what you can about any advances being made in treating or screening your type of cancer. In short, get as much information as you can to help you feel in charge of your recovery and confident about easing back into a full, productive life.

- *Understand and follow your checkup schedule.* One of the easiest ways to ease anxiety is by sticking to your follow-up schedule. The kind of follow-up programs your doctor recommends will largely depend on your type and stage of cancer. Ask your doctor about the kinds of tests you can expect during these visits. It's also a good idea to keep a personal written record of all your follow-up appointments and tests. You might find that it helps to jot everything down in a follow-up datebook or calendar.

  But why should I bother with follow-up visits, you may ask, if I feel fine and have no complaints? It's quite simple. Because cancer is a chronic disease — and a deadly serious one at that — consider your follow-up visits as the best way both you and your doctor can keep tabs on your health. In order to catch problems early, or minimize and possibly avoid those that may occur somewhere down the line, periodic checkups need to be a priority. Also, if you are still receiving maintenance therapy via an ambulatory pump, infusion port, or radium implants, your follow-up visits give you the opportunity to make sure your delivery system is functioning properly. That doesn't mean you should wait for your next appointment to report any trouble you may be experiencing. Instead, call your doctor immediately, so that he or she can determine whether to schedule an earlier exam.

- *Find out who has an open-door policy.* It is important to your emotional health as well as your physical well-being to know that you can keep in touch with a member of your health care team. If your oncologist or primary care physicians seems to be too busy with other patients to see you as often as your follow-ups require, perhaps he or she can refer you to someone more available. Remember, it's your health you're trying to safeguard, not the doctor's schedule.

• *Learn how to be wary, not worried.* Part of the anxiety you feel after finishing treatment comes from realizing that the job of recovery is chiefly your responsibility now. It is normal to feel anxious, even scared, during this vulnerable period. You may find that you get especially jumpy just before your follow-up visits. Even those sturdy individuals who never bothered to heed an ache or a pain before their cancer diagnosis suddenly find that the slightest bump or twinge sends them flying to the doctor. We will deal with the issue of fear of recurrence in a later chapter, but it is important to mention here that this preoccupation with health is quite common — and even beneficial — as long as it's not keeping you up nights.

3
The Emotional Aftermath

> Healing is a matter of time, but it is sometimes also a
> matter of opportunity.
>
> — Hippocrates

A FEW YEARS AGO I was asked to lead a workshop on peer support at a survivorship conference in Albuquerque, New Mexico. During a break I was approached by a tall man with a laconic, solitary demeanor. He introduced himself as Dennis and said that the day before had marked his first year free of non-Hodgkin's lymphoma. I congratulated him, and he smiled his thanks. But something in his eyes belied his smile. I asked if he wanted to talk after the workshop. We met for coffee, and he told me his story.

Dennis was a fifty-one-year-old Vietnam veteran. Drafted at eighteen, he was badly wounded during a search-and-destroy mission outside Da Nang. For a few days following surgery, Dennis thought he was going to die. He didn't. Instead he recovered, was honorably discharged, and returned home to New Mexico.

After Dennis finished college, he married and settled down in Albuquerque, where he opened a sporting goods store. He put in fourteen-hour days and made the business a success. Life, he thought, was finally back to normal. Several years later, however, Dennis was diagnosed with lymphoma, a cancer he suspects was caused by exposure to Agent Orange, the toxic defoliant used by U.S. forces in Vietnam.

℮ I was certain that after Vietnam, nothing could come close to that experience. But I was wrong. It was hell all over again.

I was treated with chemotherapy at the local Veterans Administration hospital and got to know several other vets being treated for cancer. We'd spend a lot of the time swapping stories about 'Nam. Some of the guys did that, I think, as a way of getting their minds off cancer. It was safer for them to talk about that war than the one they were currently fighting. But to me it was all the same. I was right back in the trenches again, staring death in the face.

Actually, in some ways Vietnam was easier. At least you had furloughs, or you could get wasted and forget the war for a few hours. But cancer's different; it won't leave your head alone. You're spending all your time and energy fighting an enemy you can't see; it's guerrilla warfare of a different kind. You wake up each day wondering, Am I going to win this one?

And I did — at least the first round. But after a few months, I started getting what my doctor called delayed stress reactions. It began with nightmares. I'd have a recurring dream that I was back at the VA for cancer treatment. I'd be all alone in the room, and then a group of Vietnamese would come in all dressed as doctors. That dream always ended the same way: this team of "doctors" would begin to strap me down on the table, and I'd wake up screaming.

The nights were affecting my days. I'd get into these angry moods and then snap at my employees. I started drinking heavily, and that made me even more antisocial. I knew I was in bad shape, but I couldn't seem to make a move to get help for myself. No one could understand what I was going through. I was a survivor of two wars, and still a prisoner of both. ℮

Dennis's story stirred up deep-seated feelings in me that I had trouble identifying at first. Though I'd never fought in Vietnam, I could empathize with the way he felt. But was it his war experience I connected with, or his cancer experience? As we talked, the lines between the two seemed to blur. For survivors like Dennis and me, the similarities are striking.

The Psychological Wounds of War

Because cancer has a grim mystique all its own, it's quite unlike the fight against most other diseases. Ambushed by aberrant cells within their bodies, cancer patients find themselves on unfamiliar terrain where the medical language is strange and disconcerting, the weapons debilitating and sometimes disfiguring. Dennis told me about how some of his fellow cancer patients at the VA hospital would sarcastically refer to treatment as "friendly fire." That reminded me of how Lisa and I used to swap "war stories" and compare our "battle scars" from surgery.

Once in remission, most survivors spend the immediate post-treatment period "licking their wounds" and assessing the physical damage done. But many discover that the emotional damage is not always as easy to recognize, or as accessible. In much the same way that soldiers return home with war still raging inside them, recovering cancer patients find they must struggle to come to terms with the full effect of their experience.

Until recently, Jesse, a survivor of acute nonlymphocytic leukemia, didn't understand why he was having such a hard time getting over his cancer experience, even though it was two years behind him. He talked about it with his support group.

& My problem has its roots in my reaction to chemotherapy. As I got further along in the treatment protocol, I was increasingly disturbed by it. I knew the chemo was helping me, that without it I didn't have a chance. But even with sedation and antinausea medication, I'd get this very primitive panic-stricken reaction, like a trapped animal. As soon as I entered the treatment room I'd get sick to my stomach, and that would make me overreact even more. I'd do all those things you did as a child to manipulate yourself out of a bad situation. But nothing worked. I still had to sit there and have them run that IV, and I knew all too well how and when it would kick in.

I'm a couple of years beyond that now, but my experience with chemotherapy still affects me. For instance, I have a lot of trouble being in a crowded room; anything like a busy restaurant or a packed elevator will set off feelings of panic. I may not show it, but inside I'm like a blender on high. I'll get all the signs of an anxiety attack: shortness of breath, rapid heartbeat, and nausea. My doctor says that it's common to have some delayed reaction to cancer treatment — but my case, he tells me, is extreme. &⁊

I know exactly how Jesse feels. Although I'm now more than two decades past treatment, I still can't enter a hospital without experiencing strong physical reactions to my memories of cancer therapy. Whenever I enter an oncology clinic, I break into a cold sweat and my heart starts racing. The smell of alcohol pads and the sight of butterfly IV's never fail to make me nauseated. Many survivors tell me they go through similar emotional responses, ranging from strong, persistent feelings of guilt and sadness to short bouts of insomnia and depression around the time of their follow-up exams. Survivors are especially prone to a rush of strong emotions before or on "anniversary" dates, such as the date they were diagnosed or when treatment ended.

But these reactions aren't unique to cancer survivors. Anyone who has endured a life-threatening or traumatic situation — an airplane crash, a violent crime, a devastating earthquake — is a likely candidate for a delayed stress disorder. Although many people appear to make a quick recovery from such a crisis, some experience long-lasting emotional reverberations that can take the form of recurring dreams, depression, phobias, substance abuse, and anxiety attacks. These symptoms may show up immediately following the trauma or develop seemingly out of the blue months or years later.

Symptoms are often set off or made worse by physical reminders of the experience.

This delayed reaction to a traumatic event is called post-traumatic stress disorder (PTSD). But the name is merely a new label for an old syndrome. During World War I, soldiers who exhibited psychological disturbances were said to be "shell-shocked" or suffering from battle fatigue. The Vietnam War ultimately brought the issue of post-traumatic stress disorder to national attention when reports revealed that the lives of many vets were disrupted by the trauma of combat.

UCLA radiologist Dr. Richard Steckel explains why cancer survivors are susceptible to PTSD:

✑ During the difficult phase of acute cancer care, you muster all your forces to pull through the tests and treatments. You hold yourself together with that control. Once treatment ends, that control may no longer be needed, and so any emotions you were suppressing — anger, sadness, fear — will rise to the surface. ✑

Without doubt, cancer does leave its dent in you. It could be that you feel changed, perhaps even transformed by the experience. You may discover, as I did, that who you are doesn't quite fit with who you used to be. As you begin to sort out what happened, that process is bound to generate strong emotions, rather like the aftershocks of an earthquake.

I've known survivors who have repressed or ignored the emotions accompanying PTSD, thinking that in time "things" would take care of themselves. Instead, such unresolved emotions are apt to grow stronger and more insistent, and can ultimately trigger depression.

"Because a cancer diagnosis is such a significant life stressor, survivors often experience what is commonly known as 'reactive' depression," says Barry Daste, Ph.D., a professor who has researched cancer survivorship issues at Louisiana State University's School of

Social Work. "Reactive depression is usually triggered by a traumatic or emotionally overwhelming event. It is, simply put, a reaction to what you've been through. Health professionals consider this form of depression to be as common as the cold, and like a cold, its symptoms will often vary in degree and intensity."

These are symptoms of depression:

- weight loss or anorexia
- insomnia (especially oversleeping or early morning waking)
- tearfulness
- fatigue
- poor concentration
- feeling of malaise or pain
- persistent low or sad mood
- loss of interest/pleasure in ordinary activities
- social withdrawal
- irritability
- feelings of guilt, worthlessness, hopelessness
- thoughts of suicide

Symptoms such as sadness, fatigue, and poor concentration can also be physiological, that is, the physical side effects of radiation or chemotherapy, and can indicate that you need more rest and recovery time. Should any of the symptoms of depression listed above become prolonged (more than two weeks) or severe, or begin to disrupt normal activities, seek professional help.

Unfortunately, many don't seek help. "Because the word 'depression,' like 'cancer,' continues to have a degree of stigma attached to it, some survivors have trouble accepting that they might be depressed," says Daste, who is himself a twelve-year survivor of soft-tissue sarcoma. "It's too stressful, and so they avoid getting the help they need."

And although depressive disorders are common in both cancer patients and survivors, the symptoms often go unrecognized or are overlooked by doctors. "Oncologists are apt to be more focused on the physical repercussions of your illness, not the psychological ones," says Daste.

Don't fall into the trap of thinking that given time or the right environment, you'll eventually "snap out of it." No amount of willpower or strength of character guarantees that you'll "shake off" depression. It can't be willed or wished away any more than cancer can.

At heightened risk for developing depression are those individuals who are genetically predisposed to mood disorders, as reflected by a past episode or family history. Daste notes that for some, lingering fatigue — a frequent side effect of cancer therapy — tends to increase one's susceptibility to depression. "Patients presume that once treatment ends, so will their fatigue," says Daste. "When it doesn't, the underlying emotional stress this causes can lead to an increasing level of despair." This can be particularly true of those who have undergone bone marrow transplantation, because of the intensity of treatment and the long period of hospital-imposed isolation.

Postcancer depression often arises as the result of unresolved anger or grief over the changes and/or losses incurred by the disease (such as loss of a body part, loss of a job, or disrupted relationships or life plans). For anyone facing such a loss, there is a grieving process involved, a period of adjustment that allows us to realize and accept our losses, mourn them, and then find a way to integrate them into our lives. For survivors like Tasha, a thirty-five-year-old wife and mother who underwent a mastectomy five years ago, avoiding that process took its toll.

& I was diagnosed with ductal carcinoma in my breasts. Other than surgery, I underwent no further treatment. When my medical team told me I'd need a mastectomy, I remember thinking, I don't care what body parts they have to take in order to save me, as long as they do. Because I have to be around for my two-year-old daughter. That kind of thinking served as a great motivator and helped me bounce back fairly quickly post-op.

But as time went on I began feeling less and less safe. For me, cancer represented a real loss of innocence. I remember how invincible I felt before cancer. I used to think that since I took good care of myself, my health would hold out forever, or at least until old age. And then I was hit with this potentially fatal disease and I realized that my sense of good health was an illusion. No one is safe; there are no guarantees. A lot of survivors think of themselves as being out of the woods after five years. However, in my case, a recurrence is most likely to happen after a decade or more. I started worrying more about a recurrence or a secondary cancer, and that fear began to take its toll. I wasn't sleeping well. I'd wake up feeling awful, full of anxiety. It was such an effort to get up. I had no patience with anything, and I didn't feel much like going out socially anymore. But I wasn't really understanding any of it. My husband finally sat me down, made me look at what was happening, and suggested I get some help. ℗

Of course, not every survivor experiences post-treatment depression. Yet even those of us who were lucky enough to emerge from our cancer treatment feeling relatively unscathed or simply fortunate to be alive, and who are generally optimistic by nature, may at some point struggle with a deepening sense of isolation and sadness.

This was my experience some fifteen years after my own diagnosis. Before cancer, I'd been an avid skier. On family vacations I was the first on the slopes and the fastest down the mountain. The physical impairment to my right leg caused by cancer put an end to my skiing days. At the time I took it in stride, considering the loss of an enjoyable pastime part of the payment exacted for successful treatment.

When a friend invited me to visit her at a Colorado ski resort many years later, I gladly accepted. I was looking forward to spending time with her. It didn't occur to me that perhaps I'd find the visit emotionally masochistic.

Each morning, my friend would trudge out to the ski lifts and I'd accompany her. As she ascended the slopes I'd wave her off, then head back to our cabin. I was determined not to let self-pity get the better of me, and kept telling myself it was no big deal.

My stoicism held out for as long as my visit, then gave way on the plane ride home. I broke down, flooded by tears of anger, sadness, and resentment over my inability to ski ever again.

I wish I could say that having a good cry washed away my bitterness. But it didn't. Those feelings deepened until eventually I was diagnosed with moderate reactive depression. Several months of psychotherapy and antidepressant medication allowed me to see beyond my losses and focus on other abilities I'd acquired since my illness.

Like Tasha, I found that I wasn't in a place to get the help I needed until I'd first recognized and accepted the fact that I was depressed. But your efforts can't end there. You must also be willing to actively participate in fighting depression, trying to understand the thoughts and feelings that underlie it.

How you reestablish your emotional equilibrium after cancer will depend on your coping style, as well as on the severity of your symptoms. It is important to remember, however, that although delayed stress reactions or depression may not be avoidable, neither can be successfully treated. Both depression and PTSD are common, normal reactions to your cancer experience, and are therefore nothing to be ashamed of or silent about. If cancer's aftershocks are rattling your recovery, grab hold of whatever therapeutic tools will best help you cope.

Tasha started attending a Cancervive support group and found that the opportunity to express herself allowed her to see that she wasn't alone in her experience. With the help of antidepressant medication and more than a year of intensive psychotherapy, she was, as she puts it, "back up to speed" and once again fully involved in the joyous work of raising her daughter.

One of the ways I learned to handle my own delayed stress reactions was by keeping a journal. The process of writing helped me crystallize my thoughts and size up my emotions. Counseling helped too; through it I was able to take care of a lot of unfinished business.

As for my aversion to oncology clinics, I knew that was going to be a tougher nut to crack. I couldn't very well avoid hospitals without disrupting my follow-up schedule and ultimately jeopardizing my health. I tried different approaches, such as visualization and relaxation techniques, but nothing seemed to work. I did, however, develop two techniques of my own that have made a difference. For instance, I found it helps to have a friend or family member accompany me to appointments. I feel reassured by having someone along I can talk to when I feel anxious, or whose hand I can squeeze when I'm especially edgy. Also, I've learned how to "condition" myself by repeating in my mind during my appointments that I'm there only as a visitor, not as a patient. As a result, the oncology clinic is a much less threatening environment for me now.

Although visualization didn't work for me, Jesse says it has helped him:

℮ I had a hard time accepting that I couldn't totally control my anxiety attacks. I firmly believed it was something I should be able to handle on my own. But I wasn't getting any better using this approach. I tried doing some guided visualizations that I read about in a book my therapist mentioned. Some days this helps a lot, but there are other times when nothing I do seems to work. My therapist referred me to a psychiatrist, who prescribed antianxiety medication. So now my approach is sort of half-and-half, and that seems to do the trick. I do what I can through my own methods, and what I can't handle I leave to pharmacology. ℮

Dennis explains that his depression was much more difficult to shake.

℮ I don't remember having any real trouble adapting back to life after Vietnam. My therapist says the stress was there all along; I had just suppressed it. When I got cancer, it triggered a lot of long-buried memories. But even during treatment I wasn't doing anything to deal with the way I felt. Like in Vietnam, I thought I had to push those emotions aside and concentrate on making it out alive.

When I started drinking and getting depressed, one of the last things I wanted to do was see a doctor. I knew I needed help, but I was also fighting it. My wife couldn't stand living with me, though. She finally told me to get help or get out. Actually, she wasn't quite that ruthless. But she made sure I got help and pointed me in the right direction.

My psychologist treated me with hypnotherapy, and that brought a lot of stuff to the surface that I might not otherwise have faced. A doctor also prescribed medication to help control my mood swings. I'm not really into group therapy, but every now and then I'll drop by a vet support center just to touch base with some of the guys. ☙

When I last talked to Dennis, he was in excellent spirits. He'd opened a second sporting goods store and was on his way to Hawaii with his wife to celebrate their tenth wedding anniversary. They were also celebrating Dennis's fifth year of remission.

"I don't fool myself anymore," Dennis told me. "I know I could have a relapse tomorrow. But something tells me I've fought all the battles I have to fight. I've earned my peace of mind. And I'll be damned if I'm not going to enjoy every minute of it."

Strategies for Adapting to Life After Cancer

Cancer is a disease that strikes at the very center of your identity. The post-treatment period is a time of reassessment, of trying to fit pieces of your old life into a new way of living. But absorbing the full force of these changes can take time. Coping strategies such as denial may work during the acute phase of cancer, but coping is by definition a short-term solution. As time passes, you begin the lifelong process of distilling your reactions to cancer, as well as to any permanent changes it has caused. Perhaps without being aware of it, you'll formulate a long-term strategy for dealing with this new aspect of who you are. Survivors generally adopt one of three approaches:

- *Denial*. When survivors choose to disassociate themselves completely from the disease. They may even deny they ever had cancer.

- *Involvement*. When survivors see their cancer as a profound life-changing experience and then make it the centerpiece of their lives.

- *Acceptance*. When survivors find ways to accept what has happened, put it in perspective, and integrate the experience into their lives.

Is one strategy more effective than the others? Only you can decide which works best for you. A word of warning: the first two approaches have inherent drawbacks.

Denial: When the Escape Hatch Becomes a Trap

Many of us have felt the sting of cancer's stigma during diagnosis and treatment. The disease set us apart and swept us into "that other place," what Susan Sontag in her book *Illness as Metaphor* calls the "night-side of life." When patients leave the hospital, it makes sense that one of the first things they want to do is forget that cancer was ever a part of their lives.

That's understandable, and in the short run perfectly acceptable. Denial is a common way of coping with a threatening situation. It's the mind's way of protecting us from emotional overload. Denial allows us to absorb painful or stressful information in tolerable doses so that we can continue to function at a relatively normal pace. Virtually every cancer patient uses a certain amount of denial in dealing with the news of diagnosis ("It can't be true! This isn't happening to me!"). As a coping strategy, denial helps us push aside fear and replace it with hope and determination, the kind of emotions that enable us to mobilize for the fight against cancer.

Social worker Julie Steckel points out that survivors also use denial as a way of getting through the post-convalescent period.

❧ Cancer patients don't necessarily stop denying just because treatment has stopped. Survivors should understand that denial is a necessary part of the progression toward healing. That process takes time; it can't be rushed. In short, some denial is healthy, as long as it doesn't sabotage the healing process. ❧

Denial offers a reprieve from reality, but the cost of that reprieve can be high. That was the message of Claudia's story. The twenty-three-year-old graduate student spent three years in treatment following a diagnosis at age twelve of acute lymphatic leukemia. Denial became her modus operandi as a survivor.

❧ About a year after I'd finished treatment I returned to the hospital for a checkup. One of the nurses spotted me and asked, "Hey, didn't I used to see you around here? Weren't you one of the kids we treated for leukemia?" I remember shooting her a look that said, 'Honey, you've got the wrong person.' She persisted until I finally said, "Listen, I have no idea what you are talking about."

That was my way of dealing with cancer. I pretended it never happened. In my mind it was over and done with, and better forgotten. I thought that it simply had no bearing on who I was. Besides, the last thing I wanted was to be known as a cancer survivor. A lot of people still view it as a strike against you. ❧

Claudia thought she had tossed her cancer experience to the wind. But years later, she says, it came flying back at her like a boomerang.

❧ It happened the summer I graduated from high school. One day I was house-sitting for a doctor friend of the family when I started paging through a pile of her magazines. I ran across what looked like an intriguing article on cancer in a medical journal. Now cancer articles don't faze me. I know some survivors are phobic about the subject, but for me that was never a problem. The piece was a debate about whether or not the five-year survival period is an accurate indicator of a cancer cure. Several of the physicians in this article argued that the figure was a bogus statistic, that five years is no guarantee that a patient is cured.

As I read, my hands began to tremble and my heart started pounding. I remember getting this overwhelming rush of emotion, and then I felt like I couldn't breathe. Suddenly I hurled the magazine across the room and started screaming and crying. Somehow I managed to call my mother, and she came and got me. I reacted this way even though my doctors had told me time and again that my prognosis was assured, and that the survival rate for my kind of cancer was very high.

I'm not sure what happened that day, or why. It was as if something inside me had given way. I'd finished treatment when I was fifteen, but it had taken me more than four years to come to terms with how my illness had devastated me emotionally. &

Like Dennis, Claudia found out how tenacious the emotions of unfinished grief can be. What began as an escape route from grief became a trap ensnaring her in the very emotions she sought to avoid.

One of the more dangerous aspects of denial is that it can allow you to "fall between the cracks" of the medical support system. Ernest R. Katz, Ph.D., director of behavioral sciences at Children's Hospital in Los Angeles, California, believes that survivors who depend too heavily on denial are most likely to retreat from any identification with the disease. "Their attitude is, 'I'm tired of being different. I just want to melt back into the crowd.' That attitude is understandable, but it can also be dangerous to a survivor's physical health."

Such an approach is especially dangerous, says Dr. Katz, if recovered patients move to new communities and then decide to "forget" about their cancer history.

& Sometimes if a survivor doesn't have any noticeable giveaway, such as a scar or other physical alteration caused by cancer, he or she might be tempted to "overlook" telling a new doctor about a cancer history. This can be a major problem for both the doctor and the patient since doctors make decisions about a patient's health based in part on the medical history. In other words, by choosing to deny your cancer history, you will inevitably lose sight of the importance of follow-up visits. &

Although selective denial is a valid method of coping with the immediate crisis of cancer, you should be aware that it can be dangerous in the long run.

Involvement

Instead of turning their backs on cancer, some people throw themselves headlong into a whirl of cancer-related activities. They join nonprofit organizations, sign up for volunteer work, start self-help groups, or find some other way to connect to the topic of cancer. These survivors emerge from the experience with the strong desire to "give something back." Because cancer has rekindled their appreciation of life, they are eager to share their insights and give of themselves to others.

Christine Perkins, a psychotherapist who has worked with Cancervive support groups, began internship work with cancer hospice patients eleven years ago after surviving a bout with uterine cancer. We recently talked about what motivated her involvement in cancer-related work.

& Once you've survived a life-threatening illness, there's a great sense of obligation, maybe even guilt. You've been given a second chance, and you're not sure why. It leaves you with the gnawing feeling that you should do something worthwhile with it. Through my involvement in both hospice work and Cancervive, I feel like I'm having a direct impact. It has also helped me work through some of my own fear and feelings of vulnerability. &⁊

People who become involved in cancer-related activities are employing a useful adaptive technique that helps them handle the tangle of emotions which the disease dropped in their laps. By dedicating themselves to the cause of helping others with cancer, they gain a new sense of self-worth and accomplishment.

It is possible to go overboard, however. Too much involvement can lead to preoccupation. You can become so wrapped up attending to the needs of others that your own needs are shunted to the wayside. Before you know it, you're overwhelmed and exhausted, and that's bad news for your immune system.

You may have, perhaps unconsciously, made a full-time career out of cancer. But if you insist on allowing it to take center stage, you should realize that other aspects of your life — family, friends, job — are going to be affected. Keep in mind that involvement is the flip side of denial. Instead of running away from the issue, you've jumped into the midst of it and gathered it around you like a blanket. Like denial, involvement can be an effective strategy for coping, as long as it doesn't become a permanent one.

Phyllis is one survivor who feels she has crossed the line into preoccupation. The divorced mother of three underwent a mastectomy six years ago. Following her operation, Phyllis went looking for emotional support in the suburb she lived in outside Seattle. To her surprise, no mastectomy support groups existed. She decided to organize one.

&⁊ Anger was my initial motivating force. I was so pissed off that no one, including the hospital staff and administrators, could conceive that mastectomy patients might actually need a support group. I'll tell you, starting that group gave me back a sense of control over my life. It was liberating in so many ways. With every woman I encountered, I learned something new about myself. Also, through the group I was finally able to get rid of my anger, accept my cancer, and see it as a positive force in my life.

Sometimes, though, I feel as if this organization is engulfing me. I'm not trying to earn karma points or anything, but it's as if the support group has turned into my life's mission; I have *become* the organization. There are times when I'm not sure where my life begins and the group ends. Cancer is now such a large part of my life that I'm not doing a lot of the things I would otherwise do if I had the time. For instance, I can't remember the last time I took a vacation with my kids. I don't date as much as I'd like, and that bothers me too. Then again, I don't have the time and energy to do much dating. Sometimes I wonder if I'm using my support group to avoid other things. ☙

Nora is another survivor who has involved herself in cancer-related activities as a means of coming to terms with her experience.

☙ Lots of survivors tend to deny their cancer, but not me. I've done just the opposite. Since I beat stomach cancer two years ago, I've kept cancer right there in front of me all the time. I'm very active in a local nonprofit cancer education organization. In my private practice as a social worker I spend much of my time working with cancer patients. I also run a couple of small support groups.

Confronting this disease over and over again has helped me deal with a lot of personal issues. But it has also created a few problems. It seems my missionary zeal is messing up my home life. For instance, my family and I recently had a major blowup. My husband and daughter told me that they didn't want cancer in their lives anymore. They said they were tired of hearing about cancer all the time, that I can't let twenty minutes go by without bringing up the subject. They'd just had it.

At first I was upset and defensive. I thought, How can they be that way? It's so unfair! After I simmered down, though, I realized that their needs were just as legitimate as mine. I *was* being obsessive about cancer, and they had reached a saturation point. We worked out a compromise. I've cut back on some of my activities, and they have promised not to give me grief on the things I need to do. &?

The approaches adopted by Claudia, Phyllis, and Nora parallel my own attempts at fitting in again after cancer. In the years since treatment I've used the strategies of both denial and involvement veering into preoccupation. For the first decade after my battle with cancer, denial served as my shield against rejection as well as protection from the psychological consequences of the experience. I adopted it not so much as a conscious choice, but rather as a reflex action. I eventually learned, however, in much the same way Claudia did, that denial is a temporary solution at best.

It wasn't until I started Cancervive that I realized how much I needed to understand the past and integrate its meaning into the present. The organization gave me the perfect excuse for shifting tactics. Like Phyllis, I charged into a long phase of preoccupation. By the end of my second year with Cancervive, I'd reached burnout. As with Nora, my family was instrumental in calling my attention to my overinvolvement. With their help I came to see that I needed to formulate a more balanced approach. One of the ways I did this was by pulling back from the day-to-day operations of the organization, shifting much of that responsibility to other Cancervive staffers. For instance, as much as I enjoyed one-on-one peer counseling, I also found it emotionally draining. I realized that if I was going to continue working effectively for the organization, I needed to establish some emotional distance from it. After curtailing my involvement in counseling, I became more focused. After swinging from denial to preoccupation, I finally reached a level of acceptance, a psychological centering, a comfortable middle ground.

Full recovery from cancer depends not only on how well you manage the physical healing, but your own psychological recuperation as well. Acceptance of your cancer experience involves a continual appraisal of its meaning as it relates to every aspect of your life. You're bound to uncover several layers of emotions in the process. Let it happen. Work through them. Give yourself a chance to heal.

A Fuller Sense of Life

"There is a time of departure," the playwright Tennessee Williams once wrote, "even when there's no certain place to go." Without knowing precisely how or when it happened, most survivors realize that although they never left town, their cancer experience has taken them on an amazing journey. When we look in the mirror, we may see our faces as unchanged, but the persons they belong to have undergone a spiritual metamorphosis. We have shed our old skins. Now we must assess who we've become and where we're headed.

If that sounds intimidating, don't worry, it's not. On the contrary, it's time to start celebrating the good things we have gained from the experience: a whittling away of the inessential in life, heightened appreciation of family and friends, new insights into the depths of our spiritual strength, physical resiliency, and courage.

For all his troublesome reactions to chemotherapy, Jesse now recognizes that cancer served as a catalyst for personal growth.

♂ Living with cancer was painful, but it was also a learning experience. I've gained so much and changed in so many ways. In those two years, I acquired insights that most people take a lifetime to realize. I guess you could call it wisdom, except most people are usually old and gray by the time they've accumulated it. Me? I've got a lifetime to enjoy it. ♂

Many survivors come away from cancer determined to make life a bracing adventure — nothing less. They find themselves reinventing who they are, rethinking their lives, and plunging into activities they never before dreamed of doing. Nora observes:

ॐ Cancer has made me much more of a risk-taker. Before my diagnosis I was always one of those middle-of-the-roaders. You'd never catch me rocking the boat. Well, that's completely changed. In fact, now I go out of my way to look for challenges. Three weeks after I finished treatment, I slapped a bandage over my Hickman catheter and went parachuting. I would never have had the courage to do something like that before. And that's just the small stuff. I also became involved in lobbying efforts in behalf of a state bill regulating the disposal of toxic material. I feel that with whatever time I've got here, I want to shake things up and see some changes. I want to make a difference. Each morning I wake up thinking about all the possibilities. Life is there for the taking, and I plan to grab as much as I can. ॐ

Since the day her denial gave way, Claudia has invested much time and energy in reconciling herself to her cancer experience. It has, she says, provided her with unexpected dividends:

ॐ After three years of treatment, I left the hospital feeling as if I was floating away from the dock without any oars. I guess you could say I just bobbed along until a storm capsized me.

I started psychotherapy some time ago, and through a hospital social worker I found out about Cancervive. I feel like I've uncovered a whole new part of myself. I don't feel ashamed anymore of having had cancer. In fact, people think I'm crazy when I talk about my cancer as being a *gift*. I'm beginning to understand how in many ways cancer was my upbringing, my education. It was the way I learned how to relate to the world. And it has everything to do with who I am today. ॐ

In the school of life, cancer survivors feel as if they've just completed an accelerated course — not that anyone, given the choice, would sign up for that course again. But for those fortunate enough to have gained a new perspective, the lessons learned are as precious as life itself.

Frances Feldman, professor emeritus at the University of Southern California's School of Social Work, shared with me one survivor's eloquent observation: "You have never lived until you have almost died, and for those who fight for it, life has a flavor the protected will never know."

4
Moving Beyond
the Fear of Recurrence

CANCER HAS a strange way of playing havoc with one's sense of time. During the period of my diagnosis and treatment, life as I knew it came to a standstill, my horizons collapsing around the focal point of cancer. The clock and the calendar continued to proceed at their methodical pace, but I hung suspended in a sort of timeless limbo. There was no past, no future. There was just me, the disease, and the goal of getting through treatment.

Once past the experience, I found my perception of time changed yet again. I was now acutely aware of the time frame bracketing my existence. My plans for the future had to be retailored around a new sense of self and a renewed sense of purpose. There was an urgency to make every minute count. Other survivors have shared similar impressions with me. "It's as if I can now physically feel the passage of time, the melding of one day into another," one woman remarked. "Cancer forced me to confront the fact that I don't have forever. Time is no longer a neutral part of my existence. I can't treat it casually anymore."

For survivors, that acute awareness of time brings with it an underlying sense of vulnerability and persistent rumblings of anxiety. The only certainty, we now know, is uncertainty.

One of the challenges survivors face is living with that heightened sense of ambiguity, of pushing beyond fear and getting on with life. And for many of us, that's not always easy to do. For survivors like Renée, thirty-three, fear of the future is a major stumbling block to moving ahead.

Renée was successfully treated for uterine cancer about three years ago. While today she remains free of cancer, she continues to suffer from a kind of phantom illness: fear of recurrence.

ঌ After my surgery I thought everything would be okay, that I'd pick myself up, dust myself off, and dive back into normal routines again. But surgery left me with a lot of complications. On top of that, I decided to call it quits with my husband. But the hardest part has been living with the fear of the cancer coming back.

I've been in remission for more than three years now, and yet a day doesn't pass that I don't think about a recurrence. I'll do whatever I can to distract myself, but some days those thoughts won't leave me alone. When that fear locks on to me, I just shut down emotionally. To compensate, I throw myself into living moment to moment so that I don't have to think about the future. But then checkup time approaches and I fall apart. How do you turn that kind of fear off?

For the last six years I've worked as a nutritionist at a large hospital. I have all the credentials and experience to set myself up in private practice, but I honestly don't have much motivation to do it. It's difficult to plan a career when you aren't sure you'll be around long enough to see it through. I can't picture myself getting old. In fact, I have a hard time seeing beyond tomorrow. I'm even afraid to start up new relationships. In my past life — that's how I refer to my life before cancer — I was fairly confident about where I was headed. But these days I feel rudderless. ঌ

Living Under the Sword

Fear of recurrence, even for long-term survivors like myself, is often the most unsettling aspect of life after cancer. For months, even years after treatment, you may find yourself teetering between the relief and exhilaration of remission and the haunting fear of a recurrence or a secondary cancer. It's a tough high-wire act, freighted with enough anxiety and doubt to throw anyone off balance. It's particularly troublesome for young survivors, for whom all the glory and promise of life has yet to unfold. Fear can limit them, unnecessarily narrowing their ambitions and focus on the future.

This chronic state of apprehension, dubbed the Damocles syndrome by doctors, is one of the most frustrating challenges cancer survivors face. Perhaps you know the story of Damocles. Greek mythology records that he was a courtier of King Dionysius, ruler of the ancient city of Syracuse. According to legend, Damocles was forever flattering his sovereign, impressed by the luxurious and secure life the old king appeared to lead. One day Dionysius decided to teach his courtier a lesson. He thought it time Damocles realized that however carefree and idyllic a sovereign's life might appear, it is never free of danger.

The following day, Damocles received an invitation to a royal dinner at the palace. He was delighted; such a perk was exactly what he'd been waiting for. That night Damocles found himself seated in the king's chair, as the guest of honor. Ready to partake of the sumptuous banquet, Damocles happened to look up. There above his head hung a large sword suspended from a single thread.

For survivors like Renée, remission in many ways resembles that dinner for Damocles. It's difficult to focus on the future when the possibility of a relapse seems perilously real. Cancer is no longer an immediate threat, but rather an unrelenting tease.

Some people are successful at managing their fear of recurrence; they refuse to be intimidated by uncertainty. These survivors prefer to adopt an attitude of cautious optimism; they fully expect to survive cancer and live their life accordingly.

Others choose selective denial as their means of adjusting. A few go so far as to believe that because they've already had cancer, they are probably immune from future malignancies. It's harmless, even healthy, to use denial to disregard bleak statistics or unfounded fear as long as you don't let it obscure common sense. Should you find yourself "forgetting" about follow-up exams because you feel invincible, your denial has reached the danger level.

You may notice that certain events tend to crank up the anxiety level — when you're scheduled for a doctor's appointment or follow-up exam, for example, or at the appearance of some new and disconcerting physical symptom. "Anniversary dates," such as the day your cancer was diagnosed or the date you were declared in remission, also become emotional red flags.

Sasha, a concert violinist, is a Cancervive member whose fear of recurrence ties in to her sense of physical well-being.

ℛ Since my breast cancer two years ago, pain has become my leitmotif. A sharp pain in my left breast was my very first clue that something was wrong, even before I felt a lump. I had always heard that if it hurt, it wasn't cancer. The painless bumps and lumps were the dangerous ones, or so I thought. I'd long had a problem with benign cysts anyway, so I really didn't think it was any big deal.

But it was a big deal: it was malignant. I was lucky, though. Treatment was successful, and I had no long-term effects to speak of — that is, except one. Even though I have physically recovered, I'm now saddled with this terrible phobia of pain. Whenever I get a headache, I'll immediately think, Oh my God. I've got brain cancer. If my shoulder hurts, I naturally assume it's bone metastasis. I was never a complainer; now that's all I seem to do. My husband calls me a hyper-hypochondriac. I'm sure my doctor is about ready to lobotomize me. I'm always calling her to report what I'm convinced are the telltale signs of recurrence. She says I need to learn to let go of that fear. "Take time out to smell the roses, Sasha," she says. That's easy for her to say. Hell, I'm having trouble even finding them. ℛ

One of the first facts survivors learn to live with is that, like heart disease or diabetes, cancer is a chronic condition. This doesn't mean it can't be controlled and, in many cases, cured, however. In fact, cancer is considered to be the most curable of chronic diseases. But no remission comes with a money-back guarantee, and cancer can be a poor loser. Just when you think you've won, the disease may reappear, demanding another round in the ring.

That is why recovered cancer patients tend to live by two key words: surveillance and prevention. Many survivors tell me they are much more aware of their bodies since their cancer. They've adapted healthier habits and learned all they can about preventative measures. Follow-up screenings are a routine and reassuring part of their lives. Sasha understands, however, that surveillance can get the better of you. Any cough or ache, any bump or bruise, is all it takes to set off your internal alarm system.

At the heart of fear of recurrence lies our greatest, most unresolved terror: death and dying. Of course, we also worry about the other elements of a relapse: revisiting treatment and its side effects, having to put life as we know it back on hold. Yet these fears are somewhat mundane compared to the more transcendent one: Can we outwit death a second time?

During the writing of the first edition of this book, I felt the long cold fingers of that fear, some sixteen years out from treatment. I had developed an infection in my leg and was subsequently hospitalized for several days. During my stay I decided to go ahead with my yearly follow-up exam. I spoke with the hospital's director of oncology and the next day underwent the usual battery of tests: computerized tomography (CT) scans, magnetic resonance imaging (MRI), x-rays, blood work.

Two days later I learned that one of the CT scans had picked up a suspiciously enlarged lymph node in my pelvic area. I knew something was terribly wrong when I was asked to submit to still more procedures, including a needle biopsy. These tests, however, proved inconclusive. After discussing my options with the surgeon, I decided to wait four weeks and then repeat the scan. If the lymph node grew in size, I'd have no choice but to undergo surgery.

Though I was a long-term cancer survivor, this kind of raw, elemental fear was new to me. During my initial bout with cancer, anger had been the dominant emotion; I didn't know enough to be frightened. I knew better now, and I understood all too well what I was up against. Each day brought vivid flashbacks of my earlier experience with cancer. Could I go through that again? And what were my chances of beating it a second time?

Following my initial treatment, I was never really troubled by any worries about recurrence. I suppose I found it easier to ignore the possibilities. Then again, I live in California — earthquake country — and was used to living with uncertainty. I could spend my life huddled under a table waiting for the Big One to hit, or I could prepare as best I could for that eventuality and then go on about my business. Life after cancer, I thought, should be no different.

Now, as I lay under the massive CT scanner, my mind raced as the machine whirred and clicked. I thought about how insulated I'd become from the reality of being a cancer patient. Time had granted me distance from the experience, but not, it seemed, immunity.

My doctor called me with the news that night: the abnormality was still visible. In fact, it had grown larger. He wanted me in for exploratory surgery within the week.

I was numb, disoriented. I needed to think straight, to make decisions and formulate plans. I found the only way I could function was to keep busy and constantly remind myself that cancer remained only a possibility at this point, not a certainty.

I awoke several hours after the operation to the rhythmic beeps of the monitors surrounding my hospital bed. Through my grogginess I could make out the blurry outlines of my parents and friends. They were smiling and giving me the thumbs-up sign. The surgery had proved negative; there was no sign of cancer.

Although that crisis is over, I find that I am still sorting through the emotional fallout it provoked. I now know, in a way I never had before, how powerful and disabling the fear of recurrence can be. But I also understand that this fear is one of the few things I am in a position to control. I also know that if I don't, it will end up controlling me.

Fighting Fear

Fear is a potent four-letter word. It is also in many ways a misaligned and misunderstood emotion. By itself fear is not necessarily harmful or dangerous. Like stress, it acts as a warning signal; it's the body's way of alerting us to potential danger. It impels us to mobilize against the cause of our fear. In its own way, fear protects us. This is its beneficial aspect. Fear becomes harmful when it is denied or ignored, or when it is allowed to grow to such proportions that it overwhelms us.

"Fear of recurrence paralyzes some survivors and causes others to become preoccupied, frenetic, or even reckless," notes Dr. Jordan Wilbur, chief of pediatric oncology at California Pacific Medical Center in San Francisco. He observes that some survivors become so enmeshed in fear that life becomes an intolerable waiting game, a kind of emotional stakeout.

&b One of the most frustrating things for me to see is survivors who have allowed the disease to dominate their thoughts to such an extent that it undermines their life. They may have won the battle against cancer on a physical level, but then lost it on an emotional level.

When I see that going on, I'll say, "Listen, you had a disease that could have killed you, but it didn't. And now you're still letting it get to you. If you are going to take on the victim role, that's okay, if that's what you really want. But you should remember that it can become a hard habit to break." For some of these patients, it is very convenient to make cancer the scapegoat for everything that goes wrong. &b

Dr. Ernest Katz, director of behavioral sciences at Children's Hospital in Los Angeles, points out that adapting to the possibility of recurrence is a uniquely personal matter; every survivor handles it differently.

& I've seen some patients finish treatment who are really gung-ho about plunging back into the mainstream. They've somehow used their illness as a way to get their lives together. Others find that their cancer took them out of the mainstream and shut down opportunities and old goals. Some of these people allow themselves to get stuck in the cancer experience. As a consequence they approach life tentatively and often become bitter and depressed. &

Few people have an easy time of coping with the unknown. As Dr. Katz points out, how you deal with the fear of recurrence largely depends on your attitude and the way you handle the problems life throws your way. By acknowledging your fear, you will have taken the first step toward understanding it. Once that happens you can begin to map out a strategy for emasculating it. The following tips may get you started:

- *Separate yourself from your illness.* During treatment, the disease took center stage in your life. You were seen, and no doubt saw yourself, as a person who has cancer. Now that treatment is behind you, has the focus shifted? Or has cancer become a permanent part of your persona? You'll have an easier time managing fears of recurrence, and thereby improving the quality of your life, if you can disentangle your identity from the disease. This isn't to suggest you should ignore the fact that you've had cancer. Just don't allow it to dominate your thoughts and self-image.

- *Don't let cancer define you.* For many of us, cancer is most devastating in the physical toll it takes. These losses often result in a direct hit to our self-worth and self-esteem, leaving us feeling less than whole. Make an active decision now to push beyond any physical constraints you may have, and refuse to allow those changes to dictate who you are. Rediscover and nurture the unique talents and attributes that define you as an individual, and realize that you are so much more than just the sum of your parts.

- *Find a focus outside of yourself.* An idle mind may or may not be the devil's workshop, but you can bet that a cancer-centric mind will find ways of creating its own kind of hell. If a preoccupation with cancer is cramping your ability to enjoy life, look for ways to transform and redirect your energy. In other words, get busy. Take up an additional pastime or hobby, or volunteer for a cause that is close to your heart. Set short-term goals for yourself and revel in the sense of fulfillment and increased self-esteem that comes from tackling them.

- *Develop a lifestyle habit that promotes inner peace.* Many survivors have found success in handling fear through visualization, meditation, yoga, relaxation techniques, therapy, and spirituality. Any one of these methods may help you understand and find meaning in your cancer experience and help you cope with any of cancer's residual negative effects. Other survivors have gained a sense of control and well-being by altering aspects of their lifestyle — changing their diet and exercise habits, for instance, or adjusting their work schedules to carve out time for more meaningful activities. Work on accentuating the positive in your life, so that each day grants you the opportunity to discover simple pleasures that you may have until now overlooked.

One of these strategies may be of help to you. There is no simple step-by-step recipe for quelling fear, and you may have to experiment with a number of them, or devise your own, before you start seeing results. Begin by asking yourself what is most comfortable and workable for you. For instance, your approach to problem-solving may be analytical in nature; that is, you work best when you've had a chance to look at all the facts. The more you know, the better you feel. That was Sasha's way of dealing with her pain-related fear of recurrence.

&b I've never been a big fan of all the New Age stuff, the miracles through meditation and macrobiotics routine. The way I usually deal with problems is to approach them cognitively. That is, think them through, intellectualize them, if you will. It gives me a sense of mastering a situation. For me, knowledge is power. I needed to understand why I was letting every little twinge drive me up the wall.

I went back into private therapy; it gave me the space to hash it out with an objective sounding board. I discovered that what I feared most was my own body. Before cancer I'd never experienced any real illness or disability. I took my health for granted and naively expected my body would take care of itself. But after cancer, I felt as if my body had betrayed me.

To start, I sat down with my doctor and asked her to tell me what I needed to know about recurrence, where it would most likely happen, the time frame, my chances, the whole routine. I don't know why I never thought of doing that before. I noticed that just talking it over with her helped me see how overblown my fear was, and that helped reduce its power over me.

I've taken other steps as well. My husband has always been much more health-conscious than me. He's also a better chef. Since my illness he took it upon himself to revamp our diet so that I'm eating the foods I know are good for me, plenty of fresh fruits and vegetables and whole grains. Changes like that give me a sense that I'm providing myself some protection against a recurrence. I've always found it difficult to exercise regularly because I spend so much time travelling. But I've made a concerted effort to get back into a routine. My husband has taken on the role of personal trainer; he makes sure I stick to it.

I still get uptight over the odd ache or pain, although now I'm less likely to obsess over it. I'd rather spend that energy on something useful. ❧

For survivors like Sasha, knowledge — and that includes self-knowledge — is a powerful tool against the fear of recurrence. Once you have a clear idea of what you can anticipate in the months and years ahead, the future will feel less ominous.

For other survivors, simply talking to those who are in the same boat helps stave off fear. Says Renée:

&⁊ I went to a support group meeting and was relieved to see that I wasn't the only person whose life seemed to be thrown off track by fears of recurrence. I had tried talking over my fears with my family and one or two close friends, but other than the usual clichés, they weren't sure what to say to me. They were uneasy talking about the 'what ifs.' There was none of that at the support group. In fact, some of those survivors seemed to be having a harder time than I was. It was a real eye-opener and I thought, Am I going to let that happen to me?

I left that meeting with new resolve. It does help to talk with people who know the ropes, so to speak. But the trouble was, I just wasn't completely comfortable in a support group. I could never seem to really open up and relax. I talked to the group facilitator and she gave me the name and phone number of another woman, someone who shared my concerns and has gone through a similar cancer experience.

We went out for coffee later that week and to make a long story short, Joan and I hit it off right away. Joan told me how fear of recurrence had all but paralyzed her after her successful treatment for stage 2 uterine cancer. Like me, she felt it was too risky making plans for the future. We also share a problem with money; it just slips through our fingers. Our view was, what's the point of saving if you're not going to be around for it later?

Unlike me, however, Joan has made a lot of progress in managing her money. One of the ways she's been able to condition herself to the idea of saving money is by investing in short-term certificates of deposit. She started out investing in three-month CDs. When she was comfortable with that, she started extending them out to six months and then to one year CDs.

She suggested I start saving money with an eye to using part of it at some future date to reward myself. You know, buy a new pair of shoes or plan a holiday, that kind of thing. Her idea really appealed to me. So I've been earmarking part of each paycheck for that. Next spring will mark my fourth year of remission, and it's finally beginning to feel like I can count on the future. &⁊

For most survivors, fear of recurrence recedes with time as the pressing problems and pleasures of daily life crowd that foreboding to the back of the mind. But because we must live with follow-ups and other reminders of our cancer, that fear is bound to well up on those occasions. Should fear become chronic or begin to impair your ability to get on with life, get started on fighting back. You didn't survive cancer only to spend the rest of your life worrying about it.

Charting the Future

One of the most frustrating aspects of fear of recurrence is the way it can overshadow your view of the future. Twenty-two-year-old Melanie knows the feeling all too well. She was diagnosed with rhabdomyosarcoma at age five. Fortunately, her long and intensive treatment proved successful. Five years later, however, she was diagnosed with a secondary tumor, a highly malignant radiation-induced osteosarcoma. Once again Melanie beat the odds, but she has endured more than forty operations as well as several rounds of radiation and chemotherapy over the past fifteen years. Needless to say, these battles have left their mark on her.

& Because I was under treatment for so long and from such an early age, I feel as if I've lost a great deal of control and responsibility for my own life. I don't remember making any real decisions for myself while I was growing up; so many of them were made for me by my parents and the doctors. It was as if my body didn't even belong to me anymore.

Somehow I managed to get through school, even with all the interruptions. I never enjoyed it much, though. It was tough trying to fit in. I always felt like people were judging or pitying me. There were teachers who would give me good grades, no matter what kind of work I did. I could never gauge how smart I really was.

In my last year of high school, I became very sick with another complication. Once I was well again I thought about going to college, but then never really pursued it. I've kind of drifted along ever since. I still live with my parents and I work part-time as a receptionist. People used to ask me what I wanted to do with my life, and I'd just draw a blank. When I tried to focus on plans, I felt lost and helpless. It's not that I was scared of a recurrence. I'd been through too much for that to bother me. I was just afraid to think on my own. When you've spent so many years fighting for your life and then that goal is suddenly taken away, you're left with this vacuum at the center. You keep wondering, "Now what? How do I top that goal?" &

The future often becomes formidable new territory for patients like Melanie, once they have achieved remission. During treatment, a patient's view of the future telescopes down to the goal of running the medical gauntlet and emerging victorious. With remission, the future looms back into view, and for some that view is daunting.

Like Melanie and Renée, you may have trouble extending your view beyond the here and now. You may feel as if you're living on borrowed time, and that investing in the future is futile.

As a consequence, you may find yourself adopting a "live for today" approach to life. With the future so ambiguous, it's easier to live in the certainty of the moment, attempting to wring as much happiness as possible from each day. But as important as it is to "seize the day," an overemphasis on today can cause you to lose sight of tomorrow. What's wrong with that, you may wonder? Nothing much, if you don't mind drifting and bobbing your way through life.

Since I began Cancervive, the process of setting goals has grown to be an essential and invigorating part of my life. I can plot my personal progress as well as that of the organization against my goals. In the past few years, I've begun producing documentary films dealing with the psychosocial issues related to cancer. Each new film represents a milestone in my overall objective of expanding my horizons beyond the nonprofit organization I founded.

Paul, thirty-two, is another survivor who sets goals to avoid dwelling in the safety and security of the present. I've known Paul, a hospital administrator, for several years, and I've always enjoyed his irrepressible optimism and drive. He believes that it was his sense of purpose, his sheer determination, that helped pull him through his first bout of stage 3 Hodgkin's disease at age eighteen. Ten years later, Paul had a relapse. However, that didn't stop him.

❧ I found that the easiest way to get through my initial treatment was to focus on short-term goals. My primary goal at the time of my initial diagnosis was to be accepted at Princeton. I essentially wanted two things out of life: a good education and a chance to play college football. Make that three things: I also wanted to beat cancer.

I remained focused on these goals and I think they had a lot to do with my bouncing back quickly after treatment. I was so busy working toward making those plans a reality that I didn't have time to worry about recurrence. Also, I really needed to prove to myself and to everyone else that I wasn't a disabled person. I *had* to believe that my goals were within my grasp, despite the fact that I'd had cancer. So I really pushed myself, both academically and athletically. I went to Princeton, became an honors student, and made offensive guard on the football team.

Nowadays I try not to think much about cancer. When I do, I use those feelings to push myself along. I use that fear as a reminder that even though I'm young, I don't have forever. I also know that I can neither control or predict the future, only my attitude about it. ❧

For Paul, working toward the future adds significance to life. He thrives on the sense of accomplishment that comes from setting high goals and then achieving them. "I hate not knowing where I'm headed," he says. "I don't want to spend my life feeling as if I'm wandering blindly down some dark corridor."

Your goals don't have to be colossal to be effective. You may no longer have the physical energy to tackle major projects. Sometimes getting through the day is the only goal you'll aspire to. While you're striving to take charge of your life, keep your plans for the future modest and realistic.

Grace Christ, professor at Columbia University's School of Social Work, notes:

&ॐ Setting short-term goals gives you a sense of moving ahead. The best way to start is to focus on plans for next month. If next month is too far ahead, ask yourself why you think that is. You may want to pose the question, "Will I still be around in a month?" Chances are you can answer it affirmatively. As you gain confidence, begin to extend your plans to include longer-term goals. The important thing is not to overwhelm or discourage yourself with impossible ambitions or unattainable objectives. &ॐ

Renée and her friend Joan used this approach to tackle their fears of recurrence and the future. But some survivors are more comfortable letting the future take care of itself. For Melanie, this approach isn't so much a choice as a need.

&ॐ Here I am, seventeen years after my first diagnosis, and I feel as if I'm just starting out in life. For instance, I'm just now getting my driver's license. I feel as though I need to do so much growing up before I can even think about what I want to do with my life.

The older brother of a friend of mine is a recovering alcoholic who attends Alcoholics Anonymous meetings. Their slogan is "One day at a time." I think that's an acceptable way to live. I mean, I don't discount the future. But I can't trust it either. I need to sort out my priorities. It's really up to me to get things moving. &ॐ

Redefining Priorities and Retailoring Old Goals

Fear of recurrence is perhaps the strongest psychological restraint preventing survivors from moving forward with their lives, but it's not the only one. At support group meetings, I frequently hear survivors talk about how cancer has rearranged their priorities, scrambled their plans, and shifted their outlook on life.

In order to fit into your new life, old plans and goals may require retooling. Paul, for instance, was forced to alter his career goals because of his illness.

ॐ Medical school is one of the few objectives cancer thwarted. Ever since I can remember, I've wanted to be a physician. During treatment it never occurred to me that my illness might affect what I'd want to do with the rest of my life. But when I applied to several grad schools, they either denied me admission or wait-listed me, which I felt amounted to the same thing.

I called a friend of my father's who was assistant dean at a well-known medical school. I asked him about my chances of being accepted. He told me that even though my academic and athletic background was impressive, his school wasn't willing to enroll someone with a cancer history. Their thinking was that a person with a history of serious illness probably wouldn't be suited to the rigors of medical school.

I hung up the phone feeling as if I'd been hit by a truck. I remember thinking, What *else* do I have to do to prove myself? Here I was, about to graduate with honors from Princeton. I'd played four years of collegiate football. I'd even been drafted by an NFL team! Who were they to tell me I couldn't handle the rigors of medical school? I figured that the only way to beat the system was to become a part of it. So I decided to go into hospital administration. Now I'm chief operating officer at a large hospital in San Francisco — and doctors are working for *me*. ॐ

Robert Louis Stevenson wrote, "Life is not a matter of holding good cards, but of playing a poor hand well." As a survivor, you may sometimes feel as if society has stacked the deck against you. Your career goals, like Paul's, may have been thwarted, not necessarily by your own physical limitations, but because of discriminatory policies. Adjusting to the compromises cancer imposes requires flexibility and perseverance as well as a dash of courage. When you encounter hurdles, find a way over or around them. That's just what cyclist Lance Armstrong did. In 1996, Lance was diagnosed with advanced testicular cancer. But he wasn't about to let the disease interfere with his dream of winning the Tour de France. Three years later he made it to France, and in a spectacular comeback, finished first in the grueling 2,288-mile endurance race.

Dr. Jordan Wilbur states that when it comes to creating a life plan, each of us has an important choice to make.

❧ You can either play the victim, which means you are going to let circumstances control your fate, or you can accept the fact that you, like anyone else, will have problems to contend with in life. As simplistic as it sounds, it does help to focus on the good rather than the bad. Of course, a positive attitude isn't going to make all those problems vanish overnight. But it will give you the energy and inspiration you need to work at solving them. ❧

When I met a survivor named Ken at a Cancervive meeting, I was touched by his determination and courage. Ken, thirty-eight, is a successful interior designer. At the time he was diagnosed with lymphoma three years ago, his illness forced him to set aside plans for a spectacular house he was building in New Mexico. Ken's treatment was effective, and before long he resumed his construction plans. Last year, however, Ken experienced another setback when his lymphoma returned. Now in remission, Ken described how he's managed to persevere:

❧ After my initial diagnosis, my doctor didn't tell me much. I had no idea what kind of cancer I was dealing with or what my chances were. So one day while I was in for treatment I sneaked a look at the pathology report, and then I did some research. I learned that my type of lymphoma is considered quite virulent and is notorious for recurrence. I was reeling from the news for days.

I needed something positive to grab hold of to keep me afloat. That's when I started focusing on my plans for the house. I carry around a photo of it in my wallet. I have no intention of stopping construction, even though I have a pretty fair chance of having other recurrences. This house is what keeps me going.

It had always been in the back of my mind to return and build a house in Santa Fe, where I was born and raised. When I got cancer, that dream suddenly became all-important. All during chemotherapy, I would distract myself by daydreaming about that house. I designed every room of it in my mind. You might say it's the house that cancer built.

So far I don't think my illness has really compromised my life plans. In fact, I've gone way beyond whatever my goals and dreams were as a kid. I've achieved more than I ever expected in both my work and personal life. Maybe cancer gave me the deadlines I needed. Some of my friends can't understand how or why I deal with cancer as positively as I do. I just find it easier not to let it consume me emotionally.

My next big project is to start a winter house down in Mexico. I guess in many ways these houses have a healing effect on me. I'm not really sure why that is. All I know is that it works. ❦

As long as we live and breathe, life beckons us to make a contribution. We've felt the tip of Damocles' sword, and the experience has left us with somber memories as well as profound insights. So how are you going to play life, now that it has dealt you a new hand?

The cards are cut. It's your call.

5
Strong Bonds and Fragile Emotions: Relationships with Family, Friends, and Significant Others

> My fiancé was an incredible source of strength and support during my diagnosis and battle with breast cancer. He couldn't seem to do enough for me. But once I'd fully recovered from treatment, he let it be known, in the nicest way possible, that he was having second thoughts about our wedding plans. Six months later, I saw the last of him when he packed his bags and moved out of our apartment.
>
> — Karen, three-year survivor

WHEN KAREN, an attractive fifty-four-year-old lawyer, shared her story with members of Cancervive, almost everyone spoke up. Many had experienced relationship problems with family members or friends, lovers, spouses, or colleagues. Several people took the opportunity to share their stories: Harry talked about his difficulty fitting back into family life after a long hospitalization; Rebecca had trouble with friends and relatives who continued to regard her as an invalid; Sonya worried about whether to tell potential boyfriends she'd had a bout with Hodgkin's disease.

But their stories reflect only one side of the coin. Several members described the ways cancer had actually strengthened and enhanced their relationships: Jack, for instance, told how friends rallied to his side just when he needed them most, and Karen happily confirmed that her recovery from breast cancer had provided an opportunity for reconciliation with her estranged teenage daughter.

Each of their stories underscored how, long after diagnosis and treatment, cancer continues to transform survivors' personal relationships. How you choose to integrate your illness into your life will ultimately have its greatest effect on those closest to you. Because family, friends, and significant others play a role in your adaptation to life after cancer, it's important that you understand the emotional pitfalls you may encounter.

Recovery from Cancer: A Family Affair

As a cancer patient, your role was clearly defined. You were expected to feel sick. It was okay — perhaps even necessary — to unplug from the world and its responsibilities. But once you've completed treatment and been declared in remission, your status changes. You are no longer "the patient." You are expected to shed that role as quickly and as effortlessly as a hospital gown. Now that the worst is over, your family and friends are eager for a return to the status quo. They anticipate that you'll promptly shift gears, rev up, and smoothly resume former roles and routines.

But like most survivors, you've probably found that making such a transition is easier said than done. While throngs of friends and relatives are feting your victory over cancer, you may be the only one to realize that being in remission does not necessarily mean you are back "in the pink."

Harry, for instance, talks about the difficulty in readjusting to his former role of healthy person and breadwinner after a lengthy hospitalization for non-Hodgkin's lymphoma. The forty-eight-year-old stockbroker found his family life dramatically altered by his long illness. Once he was back home and out of danger, his family expected him to pick up where he'd left off, to be the same husband and father he'd always been. But recovery wasn't that simple for Harry.

"We've never been what you'd call an Ozzie-and-Harriet-type family," he told support group members. "We've had our fair share of serious problems. But after my recovery from cancer, my family really began to come apart at the seams, just at the time I was feeling most vulnerable." Harry explained how changes at home, as well as within himself, made for a rocky return to normal life:

ॐ My lymphoma was aggressive, and because I developed a lot of complications, I spent the better part of two years in the hospital. I'll tell you, it really slammed the brakes on my life. Even though we had decent insurance, the long hospitalization wiped out our savings. I couldn't help feeling upset and guilty over that.

What was worse, though, was that I really didn't know how to function as a husband or father anymore. I was no longer the head of the household, the provider. It was tough on all of us, and it changed everything at home. My wife had gone back to her old job in real estate and my eldest daughter, Kimmy, took a year off college and moved back home to help out. Even though my two sons tried not to show it, I could tell they resented having to shoulder more responsibility.

My illness was especially tough on my wife, Jill. We'd always had a pretty good marriage. We both share the same sense of humor, and it's helped us take other family crises in stride. But cancer isn't very funny, and the long siege really wore Jill down. Throughout my illness, she prepared herself for the worst. She put on a good face for the kids, and I suspect they also thought their old man wasn't going to make it.

But I surprised them all, including myself; I pulled through. The first couple of months I was home, I took it easy and tried to gain back my weight and energy. My boss told me to take as long as I needed to recuperate. That suited me fine because, even though I was eager to get back in action, I wasn't up to it yet. What really surprised me, though, was that my wife and kids weren't terribly sympathetic. Kimmy was having lots of fights with her mother; she didn't like living at home after being away at college for two years. And my sons, whom I'd always been close to, were treating me like a stranger. I remember one day when I asked my youngest, Bruce, to run an errand for me. He just exploded, and said that he was sick of my being sick, that it was time I took care of myself.

Jill and I were also having problems. She was becoming increasingly involved at work. She said it was because we needed the money, but I think it was her way of finding escape from the hassles at home. We grew apart, and I'm not sure how it happened. I think part of it was that she was fed up with having to worry about me. Then again, Jill had spent all this time trying to figure out how she would live without me. She was mentally prepared to lead her own life, and then suddenly I reentered the picture. I had to try to fit back into a relationship that had gone through all these changes, and it left us both feeling unbalanced.

I know now that part of the problem was me. I had become completely disconnected from my old life. I was accustomed to being a sick person; in a way it spoils you. In the hospital I got used to nurses at my beck and call; all I had to do was push a button. After a while you start thinking that it will always be that way.

But Jill wasn't buying into that mentality. Once I got home, she had to keep booting me in the rear to get me going again. I had a hard time adjusting, and to some extent still am. I felt burdened by my family's needs while I was trying to deal with the prospect of my own mortality. All the old responsibilities, like my job, now seemed a waste of precious time. But nobody wanted to hear it, and I think my new attitude left them feeling insecure and angry. ⛈

As Harry's story clearly illustrates, a long battle with cancer has a profound effect on every member of the family. When one member is stricken, every other member feels the pain, knows the fear, and suffers the anxiety. Many families react by closing ranks and reaching out to one another. For families like Harry's, however, cancer creates seemingly unbridgeable rifts and magnifies misunderstandings, ultimately contributing to a cold war atmosphere at home.

It is comforting to imagine that once your disease has vanished, so too will any family conflicts that erupted in the course of it. But life is rarely as tidy as that. However, families that can remain sensitive and flexible to the special stresses and strains of the recovery period may be able to minimize misunderstandings at home.

At the time of my own diagnosis and treatment, I was too focused on the battle I was waging to realize how my illness was affecting my brother. It took several years before he was finally able to express his pent-up anger and jealousy over all the attention I had received during my illness. His experience, I've subsequently learned, is one common among siblings of cancer survivors. Parental preoccupation and anxiety over a sick child often has the effect of causing brothers and sisters to either act out or withdraw. A potent household brew of sorrow, anger, confusion, and jealousy, if left unattended by parents, can permanently damage siblings and their relations to one another. In fact, and not infrequently, a sibling of a young cancer patient may experience more long-term cancer-related psychological problems than does the sick child.

Readjusting to Family Roles and Responsibilities After Cancer

Harry discovered that his immediate concern as a survivor centered around the role changes his cancer had imposed on the family. More important, cancer had transformed Harry's outlook on life. Rumblings of restlessness and discontent were affecting his reorientation to the workaday world.

Harry's dilemma is certainly understandable. Postconvalescence letdown is a common experience among survivors. After all, there are few experiences as bracing as a brush with death. In its aftermath you may, in a perverse way, miss the drama and excitement that accompanied the fight for your life. In contrast, the world of nine-to-five can suddenly seem rather dull and prosaic.

Julie Brennglass, M.F.C.C., director of social services for Cancervive, notes that cancer survivors often report how the disease reprioritized their values, refocusing their view of themselves and how they relate to the world. "All the survivors I've worked with," she says, "have expressed at one time or another a profound desire to make their lives more meaningful."

Like Harry, perhaps you're vaguely dissatisfied with your job, your lifestyle, possibly even your family and friends. You may feel a sense of urgency over making the kind of life changes heretofore you never even dared consider. To make matters worse, the people around you may not understand your new outlook on life. It may even make them nervous or angry.

Because of the developmental issues that come into play, young cancer survivors, particularly older teens, are often the most acutely disoriented after cancer. All teenagers struggle with the turbulence-inducing life tasks of forming a stable identity and self-image, as well as asserting independence and autonomy. A serious illness abruptly halts this developmental work, disrupting their fragile, fledgling ideals as to who they are and what they want in life. As one twenty-year-old survivor emphatically put it, "Everyone wants me to go back to who I was. But I don't really know who that is anymore. I was just beginning to figure all that out when I was diagnosed two years ago." Parents of young survivors need to be especially attentive to how they can help, and not hinder, their child's transition back to the work of growing up and moving on with life.

Cancer survivor and family therapist Christine Perkins agrees that change is an inevitable, and oftentimes essential, part of life after cancer. Getting back into gear can, however, send you off in a direction neither you nor your family were expecting. Perhaps cancer has convinced you that you need to change career goals or switch to another college, find a new group of friends, or end your relationship with your spouse. These things happen — sometimes all at once — and they may set off an emotional chain reaction at home. What can you do when your need for change conflicts with the wishes or desires of other family members? Perkins says that communication is the key to breaking most domestic deadlocks.

ॐ As soon as serious conflicts begin to surface in the family, everyone should sit down and start talking about it. This doesn't mean engaging in a lot of blaming and counterblaming — that's unproductive. Instead, each person might begin by acknowledging how cancer has changed his or her life. Survivors who, like Harry, have experienced a change in their traditional role are going to feel diminished and perhaps resentful that another family member has taken charge of their former responsibilities. Harry's wife, on the other hand, may feel so overwhelmed that she becomes emotionally unavailable. Their children should also express how they are feeling about having their lives disrupted. All of these issues need to be placed on the table and hashed out in a calm, straightforward manner. ❧

Perkins suggests that during family discussions each member should follow these guidelines:

- *Talk about your feelings using only "I" statements.* Don't generalize how you feel. Try to say "I've been feeling neglected" rather than "You've been neglecting me." The second statement is confrontational, will put others on the defensive, and is bound to escalate the discussion into a full-blown argument. If, however, you simply state that you feel neglected, you'll be giving the other person enough emotional space to empathize with you and possibly respond by saying, "I'm sorry, I wasn't aware of that. Can we talk about it?"

- *Formulate your thoughts by writing them down.* Before you schedule your family meeting, find some quiet time to pour out your emotions on paper. The physical act of writing is now known to be a simple yet highly effective way to alleviate stress. Frequently, when emotions are running close to the surface in conversation, it's difficult to keep your thoughts focused and orderly. This can lead to angry accusations that will only serve to derail the discussion. The process of writing down your thoughts will help clarify what you want to say and how you want to say it. It will also give you a chance to take the "buzz" off any anger or resentment on your part. If your family is especially volatile when it comes to discussing domestic matters, you may even wish to communicate with one another in written rather than verbal form.

Family discussions should focus on finding solutions, not faults. Then again, we don't live in a perfect world, and few of us can claim membership in a perfect family. Should you find familial lines of communication too badly damaged to be of constructive use, don't think twice about seeking outside help. Borrow the ear of a friend, a neighbor, a colleague, or a counselor. You might even consider organizing a family crisis intervention meeting, moderated by an experienced family counselor or therapist.

The Lazarus Syndrome

It is ironic that for some families, a patient's recovery from cancer can be as disruptive as the initial diagnosis.

Although news of your remission will bring tremendous feelings of joy and relief, it could also unexpectedly trigger another round of stress. Once you are past the acute stage of your illness, family members may feel it's safe to let down their defenses, and all the frustration and fear they were suppressing will surface. Family members may react to you with impatience, even resentment, leaving everyone to struggle with feelings of guilt, anger, and remorse. Some families react in the opposite manner, treating the survivor like some kind of local hero, a secular saint who deserves special treatment. You may find family members going out of their way to overprotect and overindulge you, "stuffing" your needs at a time when you're trying to reestablish a sense of autonomy and independence.

Roberta, a twenty-four-year-old survivor of two soft-tissue sarcomas as well as a later metastasis to her lungs, recently spoke at a support group meeting about how, in the eyes of family and friends, she was viewed as a trophy.

ॐ I won't deny that even though I'm a young woman, I've been through more crisis than most people see in a lifetime. I am amazed at how I've handled it. I would never have predicted I had the kind of inner strength and resiliency that allowed me to pull through it all with my sanity intact.

Once in remission, the last thing I expected, or wanted, was for my life to become a virtual ticker-tape parade. That whole "You must be so brave" routine. It's as if everyone is looking to me for wisdom; because I survived so much I must have great cosmic insight into the meaning of life or something. &⁊

Another familiar scenario is when family members or friends stubbornly refuse to see the survivor as a well person. This reaction is widespread among people who cling to the old myth that a diagnosis of cancer is a virtual death sentence. During your illness, family members may have prepared themselves emotionally for what they viewed as the inevitable by engaging in what therapists call "anticipatory grief." Now that you are back among the living — like Lazarus raised from the dead — they aren't quite sure how to treat you. Gradually, as you regain weight and recover your stamina, your family will undoubtedly learn to stop viewing you as an invalid. This could, however, take longer than you'd like. Rebecca, fifty-five, explains that two years after her treatment for melanoma, those closest to her continue to act as if she was just diagnosed:

&⁊ Any time a friend or relative calls me, the conversation is inevitably laced with the question, "So how are you *feeling?*" I always answer back, "My cancer was two years ago, and I feel just fine, thanks. But that question *does* give me a headache." What they really seem to be asking is, "Any signs of a recurrence?" No matter what I say, how much I reassure them, there always seems to be that other perception of me unspooling in their minds. I feel tremendous pressure to be chipper around them, because the minute I appear upset or down about something, they think the worst. It's ironic, because I'm the one who went through treatment, and yet on some level they want me to take care of them, to keep reassuring them. &⁊

This kind of message from family and friends can make it difficult to let go of the cancer experience. Then again, when you have the distinct feeling that everyone is second-guessing your chances of survival, you start doubting it yourself.

Julie Brennglass, Cancervive's director of social services, suggests that you try viewing the situation from their perspective: see if you can understand what it is they are feeling and why. This doesn't mean you have to accept their perception of you; however, if you understand how others feel, you may be better able to cope with their reactions.

Brennglass adds that a therapist trained in family dynamics can make a great difference in the tenor and honesty of such a discussion: "A structured family discussion can give the survivor a chance to express feelings of appreciation, and be supportive of other family members. Let everyone know how they can help speed your recovery. Find a way to create a common goal that will allow all of you to move ahead together."

This is not to imply that you and your family should fake your feelings and act like perpetual Pollyannas. Life takes on a surreal quality when everyone adopts an attitude of denial. The key is to talk candidly about each person's emotions — the good, the bad, and the ugly. For many families, this is far from easy.

The Cheerleader Approach to Recovery

Survivors like Rebecca and Harry are often hesitant to share their innermost concerns with their families, worried that doing so may cause unnecessary alarm. As Harry observed, "If I'm acting moody, they immediately think I know something that they don't." With their families and friends watching from the sidelines, Harry and Rebecca feel obliged to take on the role of family cheerleaders.

The urge to protect loved ones from undue anxiety is understandable. However, if you're reluctant to speak up, you're probably protecting their feelings at the expense of your own, and sooner or later that's going to hurt you: you won't receive the genuine support you need if you can't be open and honest with those closest to you. Responsibility for beginning such a dialogue lies primarily with you.

Through counseling families who are attempting to readjust to life after cancer, Julie Brennglass has noted that the cheerleading impulse is a common adaptive process.

❧ One of the ways a family can begin to work through their fear is to focus on hope and optimism. But if I, as a therapist, see that going on to the point where it is excluding any acknowledgment of fear or sadness or anger, I will point that out to the family. It also helps to look at how the family has dealt with crises in the past. For some families, it's as painful as pulling teeth to acknowledge or talk about any negative emotions they may have toward one another. But allowing those emotions to remain unexpressed can have such a corrosive effect on everyone involved. Some families actually need to hear that it is okay to have bad days, to feel depressed or angry or discouraged. ❧

Some families must reach a state of crisis before they are willing to begin sorting through their emotions and confronting important issues. If you need to talk frankly about cancer and aren't receiving permission and support at home, find another sounding board, such as an empathetic friend, an able therapist, a trusted rabbi or clergyman, or an available support group.

Cancer is a family affair. It represents a challenge to family unity as well as an opportunity to strengthen bonds and increase love, respect, and understanding. It might help to remind your family that in many ways they are just as much survivors of cancer as you are. Find ways to add levity to what you've all been through. Learn how you and your family can work together to make life after cancer as meaningful as possible. Harry stated:

❧ What we went through during my illness was about as scary as anything Stephen King could have written. I know some families fall apart because of cancer, and we were close to that point ourselves. For us, talking it out made all the difference. But someone has to make that first move. Since I was at the center of this crisis, I felt it was my responsibility to take the first step forward. I made a point of setting aside time after dinner for us to talk about what each person had gone through as a result of my illness. We had some arguments, sure, but we also shared a few good laughs, and got a lot out on the table.

My family made it clear that they wanted the old Harry back. The kids were especially eager to put their fears to rest, asking me questions like "Will you get cancer again?" and "What will happen if you do?" They weren't easy questions to answer, but they certainly were valid. I told them that I couldn't promise anything, but that the doctors thought I'd knocked it out for good. I explained that I felt a lot like Rip Van Winkle, returned to find that I no longer fit in the same way.

I needed time to adjust, to make some changes in my life. My old job didn't interest me anymore. I wanted something more personally fulfilling and less stressful. We went around and around with it, and eventually reached an understanding. They were willing to support me. But they also wanted me to know that they weren't going to pamper me.

My career decision upset Jill, since she thought it could jeopardize us financially. We spent a lot of time going over the options until we finally reached a compromise. She enjoyed being back in the work force, and since we needed the income, she decided to continue working. I told her I would stay with the brokerage firm until I could figure out a secure career move.

But Jill and I had a lot more to work on than that. It wasn't easy rebuilding our marriage. There were so many difficult emotions to work through. We started seeing a marriage counselor and that has helped get our relationship back on track.

Kimmy has gone back to school and I can tell she's much happier. My two sons, however, are having a hard time accepting that their dad isn't the same guy he used to be. But we talk about everything that comes up and I think it helps reassure them.

It's taken a great deal of time and work, but I think we've finally kicked this family back into shape. We're now more appreciative of each other and the time we have together. &?

Cancer's Effect on Intimate Relationships

Karen, the breast cancer survivor introduced at the beginning of this chapter, began attending Cancervive meetings more than a year ago. The overriding reason for her attendance, she told us, was to make sense out of how cancer had altered several important relationships.

&? I met Phil several years ago, and it was pretty much one of those "love at first sight" stories. He wanted to get married a few months after we met, but I wasn't in any rush. I'd been married once before, and I was nervous about taking on that kind of commitment again. Also, I have a fifteen-year-old daughter who wasn't exactly crazy about Philip. But a couple of years later, I changed my mind and accepted his proposal. We got engaged in April and started making plans for a fall wedding.

That summer a routine mammogram discovered breast cancer. At first I wouldn't accept it. I didn't fit the typical breast cancer profile. I was relatively young, with no family history, and I was in great physical shape. Then the reality of it hit me, and I fell apart. Philip was terrific, though. He calmed me down, convinced me that I was going to be okay, and helped me get through my mastectomy.

My daughter, Tricia, on the other hand, had a tough time with my illness. Before my diagnosis, we'd been having our ups and downs, the usual things you go through with a teenager. When she found out I had cancer, she emotionally shut down. With Philip and I becoming more close, perhaps she thought I was on some level abandoning her. She resented that I was so dependent on Philip for emotional support.

Fortunately, the mammogram had detected my tumor in its early stages, so I didn't require further treatment. During my recuperation from surgery, I began to notice changes in Philip. For example, when he would kiss me, he'd kiss my forehead instead of my lips. Or when I'd talk about doing something in the future, like planning a vacation for the two of us, he was noncommittal. It bothered me that he left the room whenever I tended to my incision. At first I thought he might be doing it out of respect for my privacy. But I felt that since I was going to be marrying this man, he needed to share this with me. So I asked him if he would look at my incision, that it was important to me. He said okay, took a quick peek, and then practically ran out of the bedroom. He made a point of telling me that it wasn't me he was reacting to, that he was just squeamish. But I sensed it went deeper than that; Philip was clearly uncomfortable with this major change in my body. I knew big trouble was brewing when I tried talking to him about it. He assured me that nothing was wrong and that I was merely being overly sensitive.

At first I had trouble seeing what was happening, since he had been so loving and supportive during the "iffy" period of my illness. Maybe he felt guilty about leaving me at a time when he thought I might die. Now that I was out of the woods, he seemed to have second thoughts about committing to a life with someone he obviously viewed as damaged goods. I'm sure he was handling it the only way he knew how, by keeping me at arm's length. He tried making up for it by giving me presents and cooking me dinner. For a while that did lull me into thinking everything was going to be okay. But whenever it came down to getting close physically — well, let's say we were both disappointed. Things quickly went from bad to worse. Three months after my operation, he packed his bags and moved out.

That just demolished me. I knew we were having trouble, but I had convinced myself that we could work it out. When he left, it was like another part of me had been lopped off; my self-esteem was destroyed. My friends were always there for me, but I needed more than that. I was in so much pain that I could barely function. Through a mastectomy support group, I found the name of a good therapist. I spent months working on myself, reading books, and talking to other breast cancer survivors. That's what kept me going.

To my surprise, my daughter also played a big part in my recovery. Ever since Philip left, she's been a great source of support. Tricia had been living with her father, but when she heard what happened she called and asked if it was okay to move back in with me. Since then, we've been inseparable. &°

Cancer challenges all relationships, even ones you thought were unassailable. No one can predict exactly how a spouse or lover will stand up to the test. For many couples, cancer provides an opportunity for greater intimacy and understanding, and the intensity of the crisis forges a cast-iron alliance. But not all couples are capable of withstanding such a trial by fire. Perhaps, like Karen, you have survived cancer, but your marriage, engagement, or love affair did not. Was it you, was it cancer, or was it your partner?

Cancervive members who have experienced a variation on Karen's theme of separation report that the breakup usually occurs either around the time of diagnosis or at the end of treatment. If, prior to your diagnosis, the relationship was already on shaky ground, chances are the other person will bolt at the first mention of cancer. The exit may be physical: suitcase in hand and out the door. Or the desertion can take place on an emotional level; the survivor may feel as alone as if his or her partner had physically abandoned him or her.

When a couple attempts to understand why their relationship failed, they are often quick to make cancer the culprit. Cancer certainly may have played a role in the breakup of your relationship, but more often than not it plays a supporting role. Survivors almost always tell me that it was the state of their union *before* diagnosis that determined what happened after it. Cancer merely gives the final nudge to relationships teetering on the brink.

When Julie Brennglass counsels couples who are having relationship difficulties during or after treatment, she encourages them to talk only about the dynamics of their relationship, specifically excluding any mention of cancer.

&% The couple should understand that their problems are based on attitudes and behavior patterns that were established long before the disease entered the picture. They may not have noticed it before because they had already, either consciously or unconsciously, worked out a sense of equilibrium around those patterns of behavior.

When a life-changing crisis comes along, that equilibrium is thrown out of whack. Unless the couple have a clear picture of what the dynamics of their relationship were before cancer entered the picture, their first impulse will be to hang any and all problems on it.

If your partner has specific medical concerns or questions, see that he or she has a chance to discuss them with a member of your health care team. By sharing both the troubles and triumphs of cancer, you and your partner will have the opportunity to strengthen bonds of affection, trust, and commitment. &%

Picking Up the Pieces

What happens when, like Karen, you and your partner reach an impasse in dealing with the emotional debris that cancer has forced to the surface? Is your relationship worth saving, and if so, how will you begin to repair it? If your relationship is beyond repair, what can you do to take care of yourself? Therapist Christine Perkins offers this advice:

- *Talk it out.* The word *crisis* means a turning point, a crucial time, a moment of opportunity. For a crisis like cancer to be the catalyst for a stronger, more loving relationship, the lines of communication need to be open and in working order. Your partner is probably just as apprehensive about the future as you are. But if you let it, that fear will wear away at your ability to communicate openly and honestly. If you've allowed that to happen, speak up. Evaluate the changes that have taken place in your relationship by verbally confronting them.

• *Grieve for your losses.* Before someone like Karen can mourn the loss of her fiancé, she needs to work through her grief over the loss of her breast. When a body part is diminished by or sacrificed to cancer, the loss can be extraordinarily difficult to work through. When you lose the love and trust of a loved one on top of that, you may respond by turning that second loss inward and feeling somehow responsible for it. Don't let that happen. Avoid taking on the additional emotional burdens of guilt and anger. You don't need them, and you don't deserve them.

The process of grieving enables us to come to terms with any significant loss that is beyond our control to retrieve. The seminal work of the psychiatrist Elisabeth Kübler-Ross has allowed mental health professionals to recognize the five stages of the grief process: denial, anger, bargaining, depression, and acceptance. Not everyone experiences these stages in this specific order, and you may dwell in one stage longer than in others. Take all the time you need to work through the emotions connected to your losses. And don't feel you have to do it alone.

• *Take a look at yourself.* Sexuality is intrinsic to our identity as adults. Both self-esteem and body image — how we see our physical selves — underlie and ultimately nurture our sense of sexuality. Through therapy, Karen learned that the physical changes brought about by cancer in turn significantly damaged her sense of self-worth. Losing a breast left her feeling disfigured, less of a woman, and therefore short on sex appeal. Viewing yourself as less than lovable has its consequences, and it is bound to produce anger and fear, self-reproach, and depression. Don't let your losses define you or dictate how you feel about yourself. Find some means of evaluating what has occurred and work at rebuilding a positive self-image. Take whatever steps you need, such as reconstructive surgery, hormonal therapy, or grief counseling, to reassemble your sense of self in a way that satisfies you.

• *Discover new ways to foster intimacy.* We all need confirmation of our significance and worth, and never more so than after cancer. And yet you and your partner may feel awkward, nervous, and frightened about resuming sexual relations. Perhaps your libido has been affected by treatment. Accept the fact that it could take a while before your sexual life is back to where it once was. In the meantime, express your concerns and find ways to understand each other's sexual needs.

Initially, your partner may hesitate to initiate sex, fearful of the possibility of rejection or of causing you discomfort or pain. Unless these concerns are communicated, you may end up interpreting such hesitation as rejection or proof of undesirability. It's still difficult, of course, for most people to talk openly and frankly about their sexuality. If the two of you are skittish about discussing sex, try instead to write down your thoughts and exchange notes. That may at least get the ball rolling. Whatever you do, don't bring your problems to bed with you. A sensitive subject like sex should be discussed in a nonthreatening context, away from the bedroom.

You might find that professional counseling helps accelerate the process of sifting through the more complex and formidable issues, such as low self-esteem and fear of intimacy. Some survivors find it's easier to start that process by interacting with people who share your emotions and experiences in a support group.

• *Remember that it takes two to tango.* As you attempt to alleviate the strains in your intimate relationship, ask yourself, "Could I be contributing to the problem?" You'd be surprised how often couples overlook this question. For instance, you could be placing a great deal of stress on your significant other if you've allowed yourself to make a "career" out of cancer. One Cancervive member illustrated this point when he revealed how he had used his disease as a trump card whenever his wife disagreed with him on an important issue. "I would remind her that I was, after all, living on borrowed time," he says. "Even though I'd been in remission for two years, I still felt that way. Understandably, she was fed up with that excuse."

Also, it is possible that, without even being aware of it, you are sending mixed signals to your mate, signals that will alienate the two of you. A Cancervive member who had undergone a mastectomy felt so ashamed of her body that she would dress in the closet, out of sight of her husband. He, for his part, interpreted her behavior as a sign that she wasn't interested in sex anymore, and so he stopped making overtures. This in turn confirmed her worst suspicion that her husband no longer found her desirable. Since the two of them were uneasy about addressing the issue, the game of second-guessing continued until one day they found themselves talking about divorce over morning coffee.

It is dangerous in any relationship to presume the other person's thoughts. Don't make assumptions: ask! And be sensitive to how your own actions and attitude may be affecting the relationship.

- *Give it time.* The process of healing a relationship isn't necessarily going to happen with a quick discussion and a good night's sleep. You and your mate may have different styles of coping, and the rates at which you adjust to life after cancer will undoubtedly be different. Respect those differences and try to stay flexible to each other's needs.

- *Learn to let go.* Not all damaged relationships can be repaired. A serious illness like cancer dramatically throws a couple's dysfunctional behavior patterns into sharp focus. Your partner may be unwilling or unable to continue working on the relationship. And when all is said and done, that could be a blessing in disguise. Many survivors have reported that their illness gave them the space to let go of unhappy and unproductive relationships. However, don't make the mistake of shouldering all the responsibility. It's comforting to think that if you try just a little harder you can remake your mate's attitude or behavior. But don't bet on it. The only person you can effectively change is yourself. Let go of those things you can't control, and instead focus that energy on rebuilding your own sense of wellness.

Cancer's Effect on Friendships

When cancer slams into your life, your friends are among the first to feel the shock waves. Like buildings shuddering in an earthquake, friendships will undergo a rough-and-tumble test of their strength and durability. Some relationships will come through the trauma no worse for wear; some may even be reinforced, whereas others will have collapsed or crumbled.

Your friends will be recalibrating their perceptions of you as a survivor. At first they may not know how to react. A few may be so apprehensive about saying the wrong thing that they find it easier to stay away. You in turn will be sifting through your own perceptions of who your real friends are. One of the more difficult decisions you face as a survivor is determining whether or not to salvage damaged friendships. Should you try to repair them? If so, what is the best way to go about it? And if you're single and dating, what part should cancer play in courtship?

These are some of the questions Sonya brought to a recent Cancervive meeting. The vivacious twenty-four-year-old college student says she was unsure of how to deal with the friends who had dropped away during her battle with Hodgkin's disease two years before. Sonya also worries about revealing her medical history to potential boyfriends.

ॐ When I was first diagnosed, I had some pretty disappointing experiences with friends. I wouldn't have thought so in this day and age, but it seems some people continue to have a lot of misconceptions about cancer. There remains some of that old "diagnosis equals death" mentality, and so they act as if I'm this doomed person. I remember telling one date about my illness. I explained how I'd had Hodgkin's disease, and at first he seemed very curious about it. When I told him it was a form of cancer, he got totally weird and immediately wanted to know if it was contagious. Sometimes I wonder under what rock some of these people have been hiding.

There are times when I feel disassociated from the social life I used to know. The tough part is deciding how to deal with it out there in the dating world. I worry about whether I should put myself on the line, whether it's worth risking rejection. But then I start thinking: why should I stay silent, as if I'm hiding some dirty little secret. &?

Unlike family members, your friends have no obligation, no sense of familial duty, to see you through the hardships of treatment. Their involvement in your life is strictly voluntary. A crisis like cancer is oftentimes a litmus test of friendship, separating true-blue friends from the fair-weather variety.

Cancervive members frequently talk about how, years after diagnosis, their cancer history continues to set them apart socially. Sometimes this sense of isolation is due to rejection by cancerphobic people, but it can also be self-imposed. Cancer has changed who you are and how you view others, and you may no longer relate to old friends in the same way. A weeding-out process takes place as you decide which friendships still hold meaning for you. Says Cancervive's social services director Julie Brennglass:

&? It's not at all unusual to reassess social relationships after a serious illness. In some instances, friendships don't survive the strain of diagnosis or treatment. As one survivor at a support group put it, "I am a high maintenance friend right now. I hope I am not always this needy, but for now, this is who I am." This survivor felt that he didn't have the confidence and resiliency he once did to pursue friendships. &?

You may find the positive social reinforcement you need at support groups or with one or two faithful friends. But what can you do about the people who let you down or abandoned you?

Start by attempting to analyze what caused your friend to behave in such an unfriendly way. People who harbor irrational fears of cancer are likely to shun you if only because they are unsure of how to act or what to say. Your illness may also be an unwelcome reminder of their own mortality. For these people, it's easier to avoid you than to be reminded of such fundamental fears.

Renegotiating Friendships

Unless you happen to have a flair for diplomacy, it can be difficult to reconcile with an estranged friend. Pride, anger, and disappointment may overwhelm any thoughts you have of reconciliation. And yet, underneath it all you may feel a strong tug of regret, and with it, the need or desire to reestablish contact. Should you decide to try salvaging a damaged friendship, Christine Perkins offers the following advice:

- *Try not to hold a grudge.* All friendships require give and take; if your friend has given you a hard time during your illness, try not to take it to heart. When cancer is involved, you can bet that the person is reacting to the disease, not to you.

- *Reevaluate the relationship.* Is the friendship worth preserving? If so, why? Do you still have common interests? For instance, a few of your companions may be avid partygoers. But if partying is no longer a high priority for you, then you and your friends may choose to go your separate ways. Take the time to weigh the strengths and weaknesses of the relationships you want to reestablish. Ask yourself what it is that you are looking for in a friend. Be as realistic and honest as you can, and let that answer be your guide.

- *Take the initiative.* If you've decided the friendship is worth maintaining, be prepared to make the first move. Your friend may need to know where you stand before approaching you. So make a phone call or drop a letter in the mail. However you make your overture, try not to let anger interfere with it.

- *Begin a dialogue.* Your first impulse may be to ask your friend what happened. Don't be surprised if an answer isn't immediately forthcoming. Most people have a hard time expressing their deepest emotions, particularly when it concerns an issue as fear-laden as cancer. First allow your friends to come to terms with their feelings, then give them the time and space to express themselves.

  Talk about what has changed in your relationship and what if anything you think needs to change. Urge your friends to ask questions about your experience with cancer. This not only breaks the ice but also gives you a chance to clear up any misconceptions they may have. You might find your companions are reluctant to raise the subject, fearing it will stir up unpleasant memories for you. Be open with them about how much you want to share.

- *Offer the gift of forgiveness.* To err is human, to forgive divine. We all make mistakes, but many of us aren't so quick to grant absolution. Any residue of disappointment, anger, or resentment, if left unresolved, will leave you feeling less than magnanimous toward your friend. Forgiveness is an effective balm for bitterness and can go a long way at assuaging injured pride and a sense of victimhood. Forgiveness does not require that you condone or forget what happened, only that you accept and understand it and are willing to give reconciliation a chance. It also provides a new, possibly stronger foundation upon which to reconstruct the friendship. Forgiveness requires both moral courage and spiritual generosity, and in many cases, a generous serving of unconditional affection. But then, those aren't exactly bad qualities to exhibit, are they?

- *Know when to let go.* If your attempts at renewing or repairing a friendship don't work out, if your friend doesn't respond to your overtures, learn to let go of that friend. Find a way to work through the emotions of the loss, and then replace that relationship with one better suited to your needs.

Cancer and Dating

The dating scene has always been one fraught with a kind of high-wire anxiety. For single survivors, the anxiety is heightened by doubts about whether or not their medical history will shadow their romantic destiny. Some survivors prefer to avoid the risk of rejection altogether by avoiding any mention of their cancer history. They view it as strictly a private matter, and therefore a matter to be kept private.

Others have to first learn to accept themselves before they can even think of entertaining thoughts of courtship. I remember listening to the story of one young survivor who had undergone treatment for testicular cancer at age eighteen. He was terrified of reentering the dating world. Although he'd been in remission for several years, he still struggled with feelings of shame and inadequacy. He eventually came to understand how he had to rebuild a positive self-image before he could tackle his fear of dating and open up to the possibility of new relationships.

There are others who feel that a cancer history makes no difference in their social lives. They refuse to be anything but up-front and honest. These survivors aren't overly concerned about risking rejection; if they can accept cancer, they fully expect their friends to do the same. For them, the issue isn't if they should tell, but rather when to do it.

When to Tell: Is There a Right Time?

Some Cancervive members have told me that they think it is essential to reveal their medical history at the first available opportunity. It clears the air, lets them know where they stand, and where the person they tell is coming from. Says twenty-eight-year-old Roberta: "I've become almost militant about it. If I'm asked, I'm going to tell. If they can't handle it, well, that's their problem, not mine."

There is certainly nothing wrong with being forthright; it allows you to set the stage for an honest and sincere relationship. If this approach results in high attrition in your romantic life, however, you might rethink your tactics. It could be that you are using this "first-strike" approach as a way of protecting yourself. Or perhaps you are using your medical history as a way of testing the other person. "I've had cancer; take me or leave me" is the message implicit in this approach. Try to determine what is motivating your need to tell potential partners of your illness. Family therapist Christine Perkins asks:

  Are you trying to protect yourself from making a risky emotional investment, or could you be unconsciously looking for ways to reinforce a negative self-image? Then again, it may be that you have allowed cancer to become such an overwhelming part of who you are that you're unable to share yourself in any other way. If so, you might want to ask yourself if that kind of approach is really being fair to you or your friend.

On the other side of this issue are the survivors who have found that honesty is not the best policy, at least not on the first or second date. Their preferred tactic is to look before they leak. Experience has shown them that some people are threatened when confronted with the subject of cancer early on in a relationship. It could be that you are hitting your friend with too much too soon, before both of you have had a chance to establish bonds of affection and trust.

There is another advantage to waiting. If, somewhere down the road, the two of you part ways, you will have a better idea as to whether it was cancer or simply "bad chemistry" that caused the romance to sputter out. For many survivors, it's important to make this distinction. But that's hard to do if you have made a point of revealing your cancer early in the game.

The issue of disclosure is a personal one; only you can know if and when to share this part of who you are. Most survivors say it all comes down to sizing up the other person and then gauging whether the relationship has potential for longevity. Others feel that keeping their cancer history private provides a sense of normalcy and balance to their lives. If you are concerned that disclosure will somehow "mark" you and subsequently color how others perceive you, then by all means, mum's the word. Silence can serve as a shield, sparing you from the sometimes cloying sympathy of well-meaning strangers. It also alleviates what some concede is the emotionally taxing obligation of having to explain or recount their cancer experience over and over again. The bottom line on disclosure is that there is no right and wrong; follow your instincts and go with what serves your needs.

Handling Rejection

Suppose you do wait to tell until you've established a sense of rapport and intimacy with your partner. You mention your cancer, and voilà, he or she performs a vanishing act. If that person means anything to you, chances are you're going to need to know why it happened. Perhaps your partner is cancerphobic; if so, you may have little success in, or desire for, renegotiating the relationship. But rejection can be motivated by other, less obvious reasons, and it may help you deal with this painful experience by knowing what they are. For example, it could be that your friend recently lost a relative to cancer, and news of your experience may stir up a disquieting sense of vulnerability. Another scenario might include your partner's unexpressed fears and suspicions regarding what if any body damage you sustained from treatment. Similarly, your partner might conclude (incorrectly, in most cases) that treatment has left you infertile. Fear of recurrence is another obstacle that can impede a relationship. Your partner may harbor fears that a chronic disease like cancer automatically diminishes your life span.

Should any of these issues prevent you and your partner from going forward with the relationship, it's worth the effort to straighten out the misunderstanding. Help your friend see that most cancer-related fears are based on outdated myths and misconceptions. You may even suggest that your partner talk to your physician if you think that would help.

And if your friend still can't handle it? Then it is probably time to sign off on that relationship. After all, if they couldn't handle cancer in your past, how would they ever possibly manage if it recurred? How would they likely deal with *any* crisis?

As painful as rejection is, try not to take it as a personal affront. After all, who did the rejecting? Could you have possibly, perhaps unconsciously, taken yourself out of the running? And what was it your friend was reacting to? How did your friend feel toward you before learning about your illness? By answering these questions, you may see whether the problem lies with you or your partner. And make no mistake: a clean medical record is no guarantee of a successful romantic relationship. Heartbreak also happens to perfectly healthy people. Learn to believe in who you are and what you have to offer others.

The Silver Lining

When all is said and done, relationships are what matter most in life. Through them we find love and companionship, learn about the world, and ultimately gain a deeper understanding of ourselves. The survivors who shared their stories in this chapter weathered tough times in their relationships with friends and loved ones, and each carried away a special lesson from the experience.

Not all relationships suffer as a consequence of cancer; many of them flourish. Jack's is one of them.

Now in his fifth year of remission from chronic myelogenous leukemia, the thirty-eight-year-old entrepreneur has a distinctive way of celebrating survival. Each summer, on the anniversary of his successful bone marrow transplant, he plays a round of golf with his friends. But this isn't just any golf game, and this isn't just any group of friends. Jack proudly reports that last year his annual Platelet Open golf tournament raised thousands of dollars for the Leukemia Society. He explains how, with a little help from his nearest and dearest, his fundraising idea occurred.

❧ I was thirty-one when I was diagnosed with leukemia. I had a wife and two kids, with a third baby on the way. When my doctor called me with the news, I sat down and cried my eyes out for about five minutes. And then, just as quickly, I snapped out of it. I immediately made up my mind that I was going to beat this thing. And even if I couldn't, and I only lived the two years the doctors were giving me, I was determined to make them the happiest years of my life. For me, maintaining a positive attitude was the key to getting through cancer.

A few months after my diagnosis, my leukemia went into an acute phase. My doctors were able to control it, but they told me that without a bone marrow transplant I probably wouldn't make it. I underwent an autologous, or "self," bone marrow transplant, and it really knocked me for a loop. While I was recovering in the hospital, I learned that a group of my friends and business associates had been donating blood on a regular basis to give me the platelet transfusions I needed to keep my blood clotting normally. I run a family construction business, and while I was out sick, my secretary organized a blood donor program for me. All my donor friends wore beepers so that when my doctors knew I needed a transfusion of platelets, the hospital would call my secretary. She would check her donor list and then beep one of the platelet volunteers. A lot of these people lived way out in the suburbs, which meant they had to take time off from work and make the long drive to the hospital to donate blood. The efforts of my friends and family went far beyond what I could ever have imagined. It was an incredible show of love, support, and friendship. Without them I probably wouldn't be here today.

As I was about to turn thirty-five, I decided to throw a party to celebrate both my birthday and my survival. I also wanted to officially thank all my donor friends. I knew that most of my friends enjoyed golf, so I invited the group to join me for lunch and a game at the local country club. After the golf game, I gave each person a red sweater embroidered with the words "Platelet Open." The afternoon was a big success. In fact, everyone had such a good time that they kept asking me, "Where do you plan on taking us next year, Jack?"

That got me thinking. I had survived cancer, and I had a strong desire to show my gratitude. Then the idea hit me: why not sponsor a golf game every year and turn it into a fundraiser? I approached the Leukemia Society, and that's how the Platelet Open was born. We just held our fourth annual tournament, and I'm proud to report that we raised more than forty thousand dollars.

I can't say that having leukemia was a wonderful experience, but for me it resulted in a lot of wonderful things. Cancer clarified what was really important in my life, and I now know how lucky I am to have such a wonderful family and friends. Thanks to them, I plan on having a happy life. &?

6
The Insurance Obstacle

FOR THE ANCIENT GREEKS, life was ruled by fate. They believed that each man's destiny was determined by powers beyond his control, that the course of events was already written.

Most people don't put much stock in that notion today. And yet when it comes to health insurance, cancer survivors often feel as if their fate were indeed written — not in the heavens, but in the computer files of insurance companies across the nation.

As a survivor, you are undoubtedly proud of your victory over cancer. The battle you waged was nothing short of heroic. But that isn't how the insurance industry sees it. In its book, a history of cancer makes you a liability, not a hero. You may want to put cancer behind you, but that's not always easy. The insurance obstacle is there to remind you of it.

You are reminded every time you apply for a health, life, or disability insurance policy. Before you can say the words "preexisting condition," a verdict of *coverage denied* may come back at you. (In the parlance of insurance companies, a preexisting condition is a medical problem or condition that was diagnosed and/or treated prior to an application for insurance coverage.) You are reminded when premiums on an existing policy skyrocket to the point where you can no longer afford health insurance. If you are lucky enough to secure coverage through your employer, your insurance company may require a six- to twelve-month waiting period before it will cover cancer-related expenses. Or the policy may come with an "impairment exclusion" rider, meaning that the insurance company will cover everything except, of course, cancer.

Years pass and you may come to regard your bout with cancer as your little secret. But don't fool yourself: the insurance industry is probably in on it. Medical details from insurance applications or medical claims you or your doctors may have filed in the last seven years can wind up in the data banks of the Boston-based Medical Information Bureau (MIB).

The MIB was founded in 1902 as a way to protect both insurance companies and policyholders against fraud. Functioning much like a national credit reporting bureau, the MIB holds vast stores of computerized data for its approximately eight-hundred-member commercial insurance carriers (excluding Blue Cross/Blue Shield). Member insurance companies tap into the MIB whenever they want to verify the medical history of a new applicant. Should such a check reveal omissions, misinformation, or inconsistencies (or for that matter, major medical problems) on the part of the applicant, coverage may be denied or an existing policy canceled. Call it data bank destiny: when it comes to health insurance, you are, in part, the sum of your charts.

You can, however, verify information and correct inaccuracies by obtaining a copy of your MIB files. For a nominal fee, request a disclosure form by writing to Medical Information Bureau, Inc., P.O. Box 105, Essex Station, Boston, MA 02112. The MIB can also be reached by phone, (617) 426-3660, or through their Web site, www.mib.com.

The Bottom Line

What can you do? As someone with a chronic disease, your need for quality health insurance is essential. Most Americans today find coverage through their place of employment or that of their spouse's. But there are many who aren't so fortunate, such as those who work part-time or for a small business, are self-employed, or aren't attached to a partner's policy. In these instances, your eligibility for coverage as a survivor could well depend on the kind of cancer you've had as well as the length of time you've been disease-free. Should you, on the one hand, attempt to conceal your cancer diagnosis on an application form and are later found out, your policy may be canceled and your claims denied. On the other hand, if you tell the truth, there is a chance you could be refused coverage, or offered it at extremely high rates and/or with reduced benefits.

In short, it doesn't matter how well you feel or how positive your doctor's prognosis may be. Once your insurance application is stamped HIGH RISK, your ability to buy protection against the cost of future illness may be seriously diminished. As a result, the threat of financial disaster can loom just out of sight for many survivors.

If insurance is there to protect us, why are so many millions of people left unprotected? Insurers say the reasons behind their restrictions boil down to pure financial survival. Naturally, the bottom line is important to insurance company stockholders. To ensure profits, management strives to control costs. One of the ways they do this (except in states that prohibit the practice) is by restricting or eliminating the types of people they will insure — specifically, high-risk applicants.

Who makes these decisions? Insurance underwriters do. Utilizing actuarial reports and studies, they determine what medical conditions constitute a bad or "substandard" risk. The health insurance industry is most interested in "preferred" or "standard" risks; that is, those who aren't likely to file a lot of claims. From the insurance industry's viewpoint, this policy of "risk management" is not discriminatory; it's merely prudent business practice. But to those who have trouble obtaining or maintaining insurance due to a pre-existing health condition, that practice often goes by other unprintable names.

Managed care programs such as HMOs (health maintenance organizations), PPOs (preferred provider organizations), and POSs (point of service networks) have served to tighten the squeeze on access to health care. These plans offer comprehensive medical services on a fixed prepaid basis. Members of managed care plans pay regularly into the plan and in return are entitled to the medical services of participating hospitals and doctors. When HMOs began their climb to dominance in the 1980s, they were considered to be an attractive, cost-effective alternative to traditional indemnity (also known as "fee-for-service") medicine. To be sure, their cost-cutting approach to health care has transformed the everyday practice of medicine. In too many instances, however, this approach has also compromised the quality of care cancer patients and survivors receive.

Simply put, managed care programs are the modern-day marriage of business principles to the delivery of health care. But for many health care consumers, the union has not been a success. The maximization of profits all too often collides with the best interests of patients. Cost-cutting and economic considerations on the part of managed health care networks can translate into narrower treatment options for its members. Doctors are required to see more patients in less time and may find themselves financially disinclined to recommend additional tests or referrals to specialists. In the bargain, medical trust as well as patient and doctor autonomy have all but broken down. But there is good news. Federal and state legislators are beginning to act on the public's simmering frustration over the need to overhaul the health care and insurance industries.

Since the first edition of this book appeared in 1991, health insurance reform has gained momentum on the state level, most notably with the passage of the Patients' Bill of Rights. While comprehensive federal legislation guaranteeing health insurance for all continues to elude us, a patchwork of federal laws now in place provides somewhat easier access to coverage for people with chronic illnesses. Keep in mind that change is the operative word on the health insurance scene today. It is important, both to your physical health and your financial well-being, that you remain an aggressively informed consumer. By both understanding the options currently available, and developing a strong sense of self-advocacy, you'll be better equipped to navigate health insurance situations.

Common Obstacles to Obtaining or Keeping Insurance

Job Lock

Not long ago, survivors insured at work faced an uphill battle regarding coverage whenever they needed to find new employment. Unless they could land a new job quickly, one where the insurance underwriter didn't ask questions about new employees, access to adequate and affordable health insurance often proved elusive. As a consequence, many found themselves locked into jobs simply because of the security of affordable coverage.

There are often other drawbacks to company-provided coverage. For instance, what if you are a full-time employee and, because of health or personal reasons, you need to cut back on your work schedule? Since part-timers and hourly wage earners are rarely included under an employer-sponsored health insurance plan, you're stuck: if you trim your work schedule, you could jeopardize your benefits. Or perhaps you have ambitions of quitting the company and going into business for yourself. Inability to obtain affordable private coverage can quickly douse your dreams of entrepreneurship.

Adult survivors of childhood cancers who don't have either a solid work history or insurance through parents or a spouse are most vulnerable to insurance problems. Too old to continue coverage under their parents' policy, they encounter a multitude of barriers to obtaining health insurance. Survivors like Allen often find themselves grappling with the problem of "school lock." Since the age of fifteen, Allen has survived three bouts with Ewing's sarcoma. He's now a twenty-seven-year-old graduate student in the Special Education Department of a California university.

❧ At the time I was first diagnosed, I had plans to go into the military. Unfortunately, the surgery on my right leg took care of that. Realizing that I had to shift my goals to fit my disability, I spent quite a while weighing the work options left to me. I looked for a profession where I could deal with small groups of people and have a limited workday, and yet have access to a good group insurance policy.

Happily, I've found all that in my current position as an assistant teacher in a Special Ed department. I can keep my benefits package as long as I remain enrolled in school and continue taking degrees. I can't say that I feel like a recipient of direct insurance discrimination per se. But then again, I do feel somewhat trapped. It feels like I can't move out of school and on with my life, because I need this insurance. &8

Diagnosed with cancer at roughly the same age as Allen, I faced a similar situation. My own rude awakening to insurance problems came at age twenty-three, when coverage under my parents' policy expired. With my treatment for rhabdomyosarcoma five years behind me, I didn't think I'd have all that much trouble locating individual coverage on my own. My parents were as distressed as I was to find out how wrong that perception was. Eventually I found coverage under my employer's group plan.

Some years later I came to understand job lock firsthand. Employed at a large department store as a special events director, I'd spent several years working my way up the management ladder. The salary was excellent, and I appreciated the generous benefits package that came with it. One day, however, my supervisor informed me that the store was undergoing reorganization. My position, along with half a dozen others, was to be eliminated. I worked with the personnel director, but he wasn't able to locate any openings for me. I was worried, but losing my job didn't scare me as much as the thought of losing my benefits. I still viewed my health insurance as the only real protection I had against the financial hardships of a possible recurrence.

I was so desperate to keep my coverage that I accepted another position at a branch store located more than an hour's drive from my home. There were no openings in the store's public relations department, or any other equivalent management position, so I swallowed my pride and took a job as a salesperson. I knew that I would be underemployed, but at least I'd retained my health insurance.

Fortunately, the Health Insurance Portability and Accountability Act (HIPAA) of 1996, while not exactly a panacea, provides wider latitude for those with preexisting conditions to retain coverage once they leave their job. Before passage of this federal law, employers could legally decline coverage to any new employee with a preexisting condition.

Under HIPAA, individuals who have been covered under an employee plan for at least one year are guaranteed the right to retain coverage or obtain new coverage. The law also limits or eliminates exclusions for preexisting conditions. In order to qualify for protection under the law, a number of provisions come into play. For instance, group health plans can still apply preexisting condition restrictions (for up to a year) to a new employee if that employee was not previously covered for twelve consecutive months prior to enrollment in the new plan. If the employee was previously insured, but for less than twelve consecutive months, the preexisting exclusion period must be reduced by the number of months he or she was covered under the old plan.

As an example, let's say you plan to switch jobs. At the position you are leaving, you were insured under that employer's group health plan, but only for five months. The new company can legally restrict coverage for your preexisting condition, but in this case, for no more than seven months. In other words, the exclusion period under your new plan must be reduced by the number of months in which you were previously insured. If you intend to switch from an employer-sponsored group health plan to an individual policy, you will have to show that you were covered under the group policy for no fewer than eighteen months.

HIPAA's fine print holds a few catches as well. The switch from your previous employer-sponsored plan to an *individual* plan *must occur within sixty-three days* for you to have protection under the law.

Also, if you enjoyed great health benefits at your last job, HIPAA doesn't give you the right to take them with you. HIPAA only guarantees access to insurance if — and only if — it is provided for by your new employer. Nor does HIPAA require employers to provide coverage for all medical conditions.

Sound confusing? You're not alone in thinking so. To learn more about HIPAA, visit the Health Care Financing Administration's Web site at www.hhs.gov.

Finally, a word of caution: like most laws, HIPAA has its share of loopholes, and there are many businesses that are more than willing to exploit them. Robert Enteen, Ph.D., is a health insurance expert with more than twenty-five years of experience in health policy and patient advocacy. He is also the author of the indispensable guide, *Health Insurance: How to Get It, Keep It, or Improve What You've Got.* According to Dr. Enteen, "While the HIPAA provides certain key protections and assurances, a great deal of evidence suggests that insurance companies are not always complying with it. A truly savvy consumer shouldn't be sanguine about this. Those with preexisting conditions should realize how essential it is to fully understand their rights under the law."

Of course, many of us don't fully understand our rights. All the fine print and legalese cause our eyes to glaze over. And yet, given the cost of medical care today, health insurance legislation and health insurance policies are critically important to your well-being as a survivor. They are serious documents that can have a serious, even drastic effect on the quality of your life. Seek the help of professionals, either by enlisting the advice of social workers, cancer organizations, your state insurance department, or an attorney who specializes in insurance.

Wedlock

Divorce is rarely if ever a stress-free event. For those with a serious preexisting condition, however, the emotional devastation accompanying a divorce can be exacerbated by the potential loss of insurance coverage under a spouse's plan. Shirley's story illustrates how the insurance ramifications of a marital breakup resulted in her feeling locked in a failed marriage:

& It was a week before our ninth wedding anniversary when my husband and I decided to call it quits. As if enduring treatment for cervical cancer wasn't enough, I then had to deal with the stress of divorce and the anxiety of losing coverage under my husband's employer's group policy.

At the time of our split my husband was working as an animator at a large film studio; I was a part-time substitute teacher. With my cancer history, I seriously doubted that I could get an individual insurance policy. My lawyer told me I was eligible to continue my husband's coverage under COBRA [Consolidated Omnibus Budget Reconciliation Act of 1986]. That sounded good — until I learned how expensive the premiums would be. There was no way I could meet those payments.

What was I going to do? The idea of not being able to afford insurance terrified me. Even though I'd been the one to want a divorce in the first place, I was beginning to rethink things. For the sake of keeping my insurance, staying together seemed to be the only option I had.

My husband and I tried hard to make the marriage work, but in the end, we both realized it was a lost cause. Fortunately, as part of our divorce settlement, my husband agreed to pay my premiums under COBRA for the full thirty-six months. At least that gave me some breathing room before I had to find alternate coverage. &

Like Shirley, survivors contemplating divorce should know that under COBRA they are legally entitled to retain coverage under their spouse's policy, provided that premiums are paid in a timely manner and as long as the employer continues to offer coverage to its employees.

For those unfamiliar with the acronym, COBRA is a federal law that requires companies with more than twenty employees (in some states the number of required workers is less) to provide continuation of group coverage to employees if they quit, are fired, or work reduced hours. Employees who have lost their jobs (for any reason other than gross misconduct) have the option to continue coverage for up to eighteen months. If such employees have a disability, and while under COBRA coverage become eligible for Social Security Disability Insurance, they can apply for a COBRA extension for an additional eleven months for a total of up to twenty-nine months. COBRA coverage also extends to surviving, divorced, or separated spouses, as well as dependent children, for up to thirty-six months. Coverage under COBRA must be identical to that offered to the dependents of other employees, and premiums cannot exceed by more than 2 percent of whatever the applicable premium is for the employer's group plan. In addition, the HIPAA now allows individuals to maintain their COBRA coverage after they've enrolled in a new plan, in the event the new plan limits or excludes coverage for applicants' preexisting conditions.

Keep in mind that COBRA coverage is not automatic, although applying for it is relatively simple. When a COBRA-qualifying event occurs, it is the responsibility of your employer (or the employer's insurer) to inform you of your COBRA rights no later than fifteen days after your group coverage is terminated. Then you have sixty days to apply for an extension. Provided you meet payment deadlines, your coverage will continue until you cancel COBRA or the coverage period expires.

However, it is one thing to gain access to a health insurance extension under COBRA; it is quite another to afford the premiums. Unless you can convince either your ex-partner or employer to pay some or all of the cost, you can find yourself priced out of COBRA coverage. If your divorce settlement includes the payment of COBRA premiums by your ex, make sure that any money due back from the policy's insurer is sent directly to you. In many cases, because the insurance policy is in the ex-spouse's name, the insurance company will issue refunds on claims in the name of the policyholder. Needless to say, this can make for an awkward situation.

The passage of COBRA's insurance provisions is due principally to the lobbying efforts of cancer survivor and women's rights activist Tish Sommers. When she and her husband divorced in the early 1970s, Sommers, then fifty-seven, was dropped from the health insurance policy provided by her husband's employer. At that time, group coverage did not extend to divorced or separated spouses. That's when Sommers, a fifteen-year survivor of breast cancer, began her crusade to secure protection for women who lose their husbands, and their coverage, because of death, divorce, or separation.

According to health insurance expert Robert Enteen, those with preexisting conditions should beware if, as an option to COBRA coverage, an employer attempts to interest you in a "short-term" insurance plan. Before you sign on the dotted line, take a hard look at what you'll be getting. Short-term insurance plans are notorious for excluding coverage of many preexisting conditions. Should you elect to go with such a plan, you will automatically forfeit your opportunity to take full advantage of COBRA coverage.

Survivors who think they have been denied their rights under COBRA should first try to settle any disputes with the benefits manager in charge of the employer's group health plan. Failing this, they should write or call either their state insurance department or the Pension and Welfare Benefits Administration, U.S. Department of Labor, 200 Constitution Ave. NW, Washington, D.C. 20210; (202) 532-8521.

Forced Out of the Workplace

Before she was diagnosed with cancer, Lilly worked as a freelance marketing consultant. She was, she says, "one of those people who never get sick." Instead of taking out an individual health insurance policy, Lilly paid her own medical bills out of a special savings account she set aside for that purpose. Over the years she saved and invested wisely, and she felt financially secure. But she certainly wasn't prepared to handle the cost of a catastrophic illness.

&o It happened shortly after my forty-third birthday. My doctor called me up and told me that the lump we'd been monitoring in my breast was malignant. After the mastectomy, I was told my cancer was aggressive and had spread to thirteen lymph nodes. I was numb with fear — for my life, and for my life savings. I had more than a quarter of a million dollars in medical bills the year I was diagnosed, covering chemotherapy, radiation, and a bone marrow transplant. It wiped me out financially. I had no choice but to turn to Medicaid. Fortunately, it paid for everything I couldn't pay.

But now I'm stuck. If I go back to work, I'll be disqualified from receiving Medicaid. It has been fifteen months since my diagnosis. I'm in a very critical period right now, but so far so good. And even though I feel fine and I'm fully capable of working, I'm forced to remain unemployed just so I can keep the minimal insurance coverage I have under Medicaid. It's like the system has shut me out. It's a very demoralizing situation to be in. &o

Unfortunately, millions of uninsured individuals are neglected by the U.S. health care system. They don't earn enough to cover the high cost of private insurance, and their incomes aren't low enough to qualify for Medicaid. When a serious illness strikes, people such as Lilly find that their only option is to quit their jobs, deplete their assets, and apply for assistance.

Medicaid, the health care program funded jointly by federal and state governments for low-income persons, provides for inpatient hospital care as well as outpatient services, x-rays, laboratory tests, skilled nursing facility care, home health care, and the cost of transportation to and from the recipient's health care facility.

If you are unemployed or can prove that you are medically needy, it makes sense to find out what kind of state benefits you are entitled to under Medicaid. Rules covering eligibility and benefits vary from state to state. To find out if you are eligible, contact your local social security office or state office of human services.

You Say Prosthetic, They Say Cosmetic

For many survivors, prosthetics can be the Catch-22 of postcancer care. That certainly was the case for Erin, who at thirty-two is a veteran of cancer therapy.

Diagnosed with a brain tumor at age nine, Erin's treatment included a year and a half of chemotherapy in addition to a course of radiation therapy. She's had two recurrences since her initial diagnosis and is now in remission. The aggressive treatment she received over the years has caused many visible long-term side effects, including permanent alopecia, or loss of hair. Most people wouldn't consider a wig to be a prosthesis. But if you're a female cancer survivor and treatment has resulted in permanent hair loss, that is exactly what your hair piece becomes. Says Erin:

& I tried for years to wear inexpensive wigs, but virtually every wig I bought ended up back in the box. Those wigs just aren't made to be comfortable on bald heads. So now I use a human hair piece that requires replacement every few years. My last one cost me twenty-three hundred dollars. That's double what it cost several years ago. What gets me so mad is that my husband's insurance company refuses to cover more than one prosthetic device. It's a one-time-only deal with them. So every time I need to replace my wig, we go deeper into debt.

I know my bald head is only considered a cosmetic problem, but it's really much more than that. When I try talking to my insurance company about it, they act as though I'm griping about petty stuff. But who are they kidding? Appearances *do* matter. &

Owen knows something of Erin's problem. A survivor of childhood leukemia, fourteen-year-old Owen has experienced a multitude of dental abnormalities due to the cranial radiation he received during treatment.

&? Neither my parents nor I had any idea I'd be saddled with such chronic dental problems as a result of the radiation to my head at age ten. Before treatment, the doctors ticked off a list of possible medical problems I might experience later on, but it was really hard for any of us to focus on those issues then.

But now it's hard not to focus on it. My mouth is a mess. I've had a number of oral surgeries and a skin graft to correct dental abnormalities such as arrested tooth growth, incomplete enamel development, and excessive gum erosion, problems I've been told that are a direct consequence of cranial radiation. But try getting an insurance company to sympathize! I'm still covered under my parents' policy and it's always such a fight trying to get reimbursement for these costly dental expenses. &?

Undeniably, the medical advances in treating several pediatric cancers has dramatically increased the rate of survival among these youngsters. But as Owen and so many other childhood cancer survivors know, the collateral damage in the war they've waged can be extensive. Studies on the physical long-term and late effects of cancer treatment are relatively recent and are only now beginning to draw wider attention to the problem.

Insurance companies are often the last to take notice. Because Owen's policy does not cover dental expenses, his parents have had trouble getting their son's post-treatment-related complications covered. Other survivors report difficulty obtaining coverage for their DMEs, or durable medical equipment, which many consider essential to their ability to continue employment or care for themselves.

Some laws now require certain types of insurance protection for postcancer care, such as that mandated in the Women's Health and Cancer Rights Act of 1998. Under this provision, insurers that cover medical and surgical benefits in connection with a mastectomy must also provide coverage related to post-treatment care, including breast prostheses and/or breast reconstruction and other physical complications of mastectomy, including lymphedema.

Insurance policies vary greatly in terms of the services they cover, and it is your responsibility as an insurance consumer to familiarize yourself with your plan's coverage, as well as all stipulated requirements and limitations. Pay attention to any important ongoing changes to your plan, particularly if your plan is government-sponsored. For instance, Medicare has begun paying for prostate-specific antigen (PSA) testing, as well as other preventive benefits such as bone density screening for osteoporosis.

When Claims Are Denied

Insurance companies deny coverage for medical procedures and services every day. While they have nothing to lose by doing so, you do. And yet, more than 70 percent of those whose claims are rejected don't make any attempt to appeal the decision.

Virtually all insurance policies provide some form of appeals process, whether it be by mediation, arbitration, or administrative hearing. As a policyholder, you have the right to appeal a claims decision. What can you do? Begin by contacting an organization that has some expertise in dealing with insurance issues, such as the National Patient Advocate Foundation or the National Coalition for Cancer Survivorship. They can help you determine whether your claim has merit. In addition, the following suggestions, while not intended as legal advice, may provide some guidelines:

- *Review your policy.* Keep in mind that each state has its own rules and regulations regarding how insurance companies operate within its borders, so what may be true in one state may not apply in another. Also, some companies are more liberal in their reimbursements than others. Generally speaking, most policies will only reimburse for services that are considered "medically necessary," "reasonable and customary," or that fall under the heading of "standard medical practice." (The term "medically necessary" is generally defined to mean any service or device prescribed by your physician as necessary to treat your condition.) However, definition of terms varies from one company to the next. Review your policy's explanation of benefits to see if you can ascertain the company's reason for denying your claim. If need be, ask the case manager in your insurance company's claims department to send you a written explanation spelling out its reason(s) for refusing to pay. And while you're at it, find out about the company's appeal procedures and deadlines.

- *Make sure information is complete and accurate.* Insurance policy provisions are a complex web of EOBs (explanation of benefits), procedure codes, and percentiles. As a result, it's all too easy for people who process claims to make mistakes. It's your job to review their work and call attention to any oversights or errors. If it's unclear why your insurance company has refused coverage, call your insurance representative for a detailed explanation. Ask what information or documentation may be needed to support your claim, and explain why you think your claim should be reimbursed as a medically necessary expense. If possible, get your physician to send a letter corroborating the medical necessity of your claim and justifying the charges involved.

- *Learn the lingo.* Understand the language insurance companies speak. Remember that many claims (particularly for items such as durable medical equipment, orthotics, compression stockings, and prosthetic bras and wigs) almost always require a written "prescription." For Erin's hair piece, for example, her doctor's prescription specifically indicates a *hair prosthesis* and not a *wig* or *hair piece*. Remember that this documentation will be the basis for your claim for reimbursement. The right words can make all the difference.

- *If your claim is denied, resubmit it.* When you send your claim back again, include a written request to have it reviewed. And keep in mind that in the world of insurance claims, there's some truth in the adage, "If at first you don't succeed, try, try again." Often, claims that were initially denied are reimbursed on a subsequent try. Keep at it, remain tenacious, and be patient. You may in the end win simply by wearing them down.

- *Get on the phone.* If your claim continues to be denied, talk to a supervisor in the claims department of your insurance company. Your reimbursement problem could be the result of an administrative mix-up. Sometimes a phone call to the insurance company (or asking your doctor's office to make the call) is enough to clear up the problem. Follow up any phone calls you make with a letter to the claims supervisor recapping the conversation and restating the problem. Include a copy of your original claim along with copies of any additional material that supports your claim.

- *Bolster your claim.* Along with your resubmitted claim, enclose a copy of your explanation of benefits, highlighting any pertinent policy clauses or provisions that may bolster your attempt at appeal. In Owen's case, he and his parents researched and collected recent studies indicating the cause and effect correlation between cranial radiation and later problems with dentofacial developments. Together with letters from Owen's dentist and oncologist, they were able to substantiate that his claim was indeed medically necessary and not merely cosmetic or dental.

- *Document everything.* Take careful notes (including names and dates) on every conversation or meeting you have with insurance representatives, physicians, medical suppliers, and anyone else involved in your claims dispute. Add to this file copies of any correspondence related to your claim, as well as any research or information that supports it. The goal is to create an impressive paper trail so that if you do decide to appeal, you'll have every scrap of documentation necessary to advocate your case.

- *Appeal the decision.* Many insurance carriers have an appeals process for denials of coverage. Should you decide to take your grievance to the next level, inform the company that you want to appeal its decision regarding your claim. Should the appeal be decided in favor of the insurance company, you can request an outside "peer review" in which an independent panel of physicians and insurance representatives will investigate your claim, evaluate the case, and render a decision.

- *File a complaint.* If your insurance company ignores a legitimate claim, consider filing a formal complaint with your state's insurance commissioner. Write the department a letter describing your problem and include a copy of your claim. It is the job of this watchdog agency to set the standards and enforce the rules and regulations of insurance companies doing business within your state. If the department agrees with your claim, it may put pressure on your insurance company. Also, be sure to mail a copy of your letter to your state representative or senator.

- *Take legal action.* If the appeals process fails and your state insurance department sides with your insurance company, you have one option left: take your claim to court. (Depending on the amount of the claim, it might be more advantageous to file in small claims court and thus avoid legal fees.) If you decide to retain a lawyer, find one who specializes in insurance litigation. Your best bet, should you choose to pursue legal action, may be to file suit for either bad faith or breach of contract, but your lawyer will know best. You should also consult your lawyer before taking steps or threatening your insurance company with any kind of action. Of course, taking legal action is neither cheap nor easy. But it is sometimes the only way to make a difference.

   A word of warning for survivors covered under an employer's group plan: when it comes to taking legal action against an insurance company, recent court decisions have stacked the deck against policyholders. Under a law passed in 1974 known as ERISA (the Employee Retirement and Income Security Act), courts have ruled that plaintiffs filing suit against insurance companies can only attempt to recover the benefits lost. In other words, if the suit is successful, plaintiffs are limited to collecting the amount owed by the health care provider (they cannot win damages). Lawyers' fees in such cases are awarded at the judge's discretion, so proceed at your own risk.

• *Be persistent.* No one enjoys battling bureaucracies, but the truth is, in the matter of insurance claims, victory often goes to the pests. Don't let the paperwork or the doublespeak frustrate or overwhelm you.

Navigating the Insurance Obstacle

Insurance companies are not known for their flexibility. Once underwriters have decided how they're going to rate you, they have a hard time changing their minds. Even if your cancer is five or more years in the past, the insurance industry may act as if you were diagnosed yesterday. As a consequence, your chances of obtaining coverage through an individual or small-company health plan may be slim, but not necessarily impossible.

Survivors should remember that the insurance industry is regulated on a state-by-state basis. Each state has its own department of insurance, and the rules and regulations that apply in one state are often quite different from those in another state. The policies and practices of insurance companies are just as varied. There are no across-the-board answers when it comes to locating coverage. But there are a few general strategies you might find helpful. Here's how you can best weave your way through the insurance obstacle course.

Get a Job

For survivors, landing a job in a large company is often the easiest way of gaining access to health insurance since (in many states) businesses with more than twenty workers are required by law to provide employees with health benefits. Also, most group plans offer comprehensive (covering all illnesses) and catastrophic coverage, a must for survivors. Some businesses have "guaranteed issue" plans in which individual underwriting doesn't apply, and therefore no medical questions are asked of applicants. If the plan does require an evaluation of applicants, it's possible that your preexisting condition will be excluded from coverage for a designated waiting period, anywhere from two months to a year. Remember that the bigger the company, the greater the chance of job mobility within the company.

A word of caution: because of the rising cost of insurance, more companies are beginning to "self-insure." That is, instead of relying on an outside indemnity plan, these businesses pay for their employee health benefits themselves. Under the 1974 federal law ERISA, companies that self-insure are exempt from having to follow state insurance laws and regulations that govern commercial insurers. This means that plan members with grievances must look to federal regulation for relief.

According to Nancy Davenport-Ennis, executive director of the National Patient Advocate Foundation, the prominence today of ERISA coverage shouldn't be underestimated: "Today, 79 percent of Americans are in one form or another of an ERISA-controlled plan, compared with only 4 percent in 1974, when the law was first enacted."

ERISA does, however, prohibit employers with self-insured plans from discriminating against an employee regarding insurance benefits. As an example, let's say an employer, fearful that an employee (or a member of the employee's family) with a serious medical condition will either deplete the company's benefit funds or drive up premiums, decides to either dismiss that employee or curtail his or her health benefits. Either action would be in violation of ERISA, and would provide the employee with legal grounds for filing a lawsuit against the employer.

The Health Insurance Portability and Accountability Act (HIPAA) offers further protection to those covered under self-funded plans. Under HIPAA, employers cannot decline to renew coverage to an employee on the basis of a preexisting condition or disability. In addition, employers with self-insured plans must notify employees of any significant changes or reduction in plan benefits within sixty days. Since self-insured health plans vary greatly in how they are structured and the benefits they offer, it is wise to thoroughly review plan provisions before signing on.

If you work for a company with an ERISA-controlled plan and encounter a problem with your insurance coverage, you may have a difficult time getting the problem resolved. Should your attempt at appeal with the plan's administrator fail, you'll need to take up your case with the Pension and Welfare Benefits Administration of the U.S. Department of Labor. Failing that, it's up to you and an attorney.

What should you do if you are changing jobs? Before you make your move, learn what benefits you'll have at your new job and if the group policy requires a waiting period for new employees. Examine your old policy for any conversion options or extensions that will cover you during this waiting period. Also, make it a point to inquire about the company's benefit package when you interview for a new job. Ask if it's possible to look at a copy of the master policy, to see what the fine print states. But be sure to inquire about specifics only *after* you've been offered the position. After all, your employer wants to think that your primary interest is in the job, not the benefits.

Locate an Independent Broker

If you are self-employed, or you can't get insurance coverage through work, an independent insurance broker may be able to locate a reasonable insurance package for you. Seek out an agent who specializes in finding policies for high-risk individuals. But keep in mind that agents and brokers earn their commissions from insurance companies, not applicants. Let the buyer beware. Agents most often have your best interest at heart when they suggest an insurance plan, but be sure that it's the right plan for you. Educate yourself by asking questions and getting multiple estimates. If necessary, talk to either a lawyer specializing in insurance or an independent insurance consultant, someone who will thoroughly research the market and then negotiate your application with underwriters.

When it comes to filling out an insurance form, all too often survivors will simply check off the box marked "cancer" without qualifying what type and stage of malignancy it was or how long they have been disease-free. To be sure, insurance forms leave little room for elaboration about a medical condition. But what if your bout with cervical cancer was seven years ago, and since then you've been treatment-free and in excellent health? That information could change the odds on your chances. How do you call attention to it? Have your agent attach a letter to the application indicating your present state of health. Include a note from your physician as well as any medical records that will support your agent's letter. This information will allow the underwriter to have a clearer and more complete understanding of your health status. While this approach won't guarantee your success in finding coverage, in some instances it can make a difference.

Tips for Filling Out an Application

Too many consumers meekly accept whatever judgment the insurance company passes on them. But what is an insurance application? It is the basis of a contract between you and the insurance company. And contracts are always negotiable. Keep in mind these points of negotiation when it comes time to fill out the application:

- *Ask your agent for a list of the company's underwriting rules.* Before you fill out an application, try answering this question: Do I know how this insurance company is likely to rate me? You'll know where you stand long before you've filled out the application if you review the underwriting policy. You might think checking on the company this way is a bit sneaky, but it is perfectly within your rights to do so. And you do want to present yourself in the best possible light, don't you?

- *Don't volunteer unrelated information.* Some survivors view their victory over cancer as a badge of courage, and as a result they end up divulging superfluous details. Try to refrain from doing so; it may confuse the underwriter and jeopardize your chances of securing coverage.

- *Get a physical examination.* If your agent thinks it will improve your chances, agree to take a physical examination and submit the results to the insurance company. Use whatever ammunition you have at your disposal. The processing of insurance applications is a high-volume business. Unless you call attention to special circumstances regarding your health, your application is apt to be treated in assembly-line fashion.

- *Don't take no for an answer.* Every insurance company has an appeals process. If you think you weren't given a fair shake, get in touch with your agent and ask to appeal the underwriter's decision. Although one underwriter refused your application, that doesn't mean they all will. Insurance underwriters vary in their requirements, depending on the applicant's status and the insurer's risk capacity. Once your broker finds an insurance company that will take you, learn if the company is financially sound and has a reputable service record. Look in *Best's Insurance Reports: Life/Health,* published annually by the A. M. Best Company and available in most public libraries.

- *Steer clear of "cancer insurance."* Be wary of anyone trying to sell you cancer insurance, also known as "dread disease" insurance. As alluring as this kind of policy may sound, it often comes with a high price tag and has a poor return on claims. Again, as with any policy, closely examine the policy provisions; you may not like what you find. Hospital coverage is often inadequate and may not include cancer-related costs, such as any illnesses or side effects caused by treatment. Also, these policies usually come with strict limits on how much the company will pay for cancer treatment. Because of the highly dubious nature of these policies, cancer insurance is now banned in several states.

Risk Pools

Another insurance alternative includes state-mandated risk pools. Twenty-eight states now offer comprehensive health insurance programs to people who cannot otherwise obtain insurance because of health history or a preexisting condition. Risk pools are created by state legislation, which requires all insurance companies and health maintenance organizations operating within the state to pool their resources and provide comprehensive coverage to high-risk individuals. One of the participating organizations is then appointed to administer the pool and is responsible for handling all the paperwork, including applications, premiums, and benefits. But not just anyone can join a pool. You can qualify for coverage only if you are a resident of a state that offers risk pool insurance.

Unlike commercial carriers, state risk pools are virtually equal in what they offer policyholders. Most pools provide for lifetime maximum benefits ranging from $500,000 to $1 million as well as a choice of deductibles and an 80/20 coinsurance provision (that is, after the deductible is met the pool pays 80 percent of your medical bills and you pay the remaining 20 percent up to a designated maximum. If your expenses go higher than this maximum, the pool will cover 100 percent). While risk pools offer fairly comprehensive core benefits, coverage can be skimpy for auxiliary items such as durable medical equipment and maintenance physical therapy or occupational therapy. Many pools also require a waiting period of up to six months for preexisting conditions.

The drawback to risk pool insurance is the price tag. Depending on the state, risk pool premiums can run as much as 125 percent higher than what comparable coverage would cost a standard-risk applicant. Although these premiums are by no means cheap, risk pools do offer another option for those who have been denied health insurance because of a preexisting condition. Call your state insurance department or commissioner to find out what may be available in your state, as well as any rules of eligibility that may apply. Should you need assistance locating the right office, contact the National Association of Insurance Commissioners (see the listing under Resources for Insurance Information at the end of this chapter).

Blue Cross/Blue Shield Associations

In several states, Blue Cross/Blue Shield offers biannual open enrollment periods (usually in the spring and fall), when high-risk applicants are accepted regardless of their medical history. However, many of these plans require a waiting period (from six months to one year) before they will cover you for a preexisting condition. As with risk pool insurance, premiums for the "Blues" plans are high and vary from one plan to another. Periods of open enrollment also vary from state to state. For further information, check with your local Blue Cross/Blue Shield company or call your state insurance department.

Join a Group or an Association

You've never been a joiner? It could make a difference in your search for insurance. Many professional, fraternal, civic, and trade organizations offer group insurance to their members. If you are a college alumnus, why not join your alumni association? If you're age fifty or older, look into the American Association of Retired Persons. Organizations like these frequently offer health plans to their members, some of which don't require medical underwriting.

How do you go about tracking down such an organization? To start, make a trip to the reference section of your library and ask for a book called the *Encyclopedia of Associations*. Look up the organizations that most appeal to you. Then contact them to find out the kind of insurance, if any, they offer members. But caveat emptor. Some of these plans are better than others, and premiums can vary dramatically. While you are shopping around, remember to look for a plan that offers comprehensive coverage.

The Need for National Health Insurance

The American system of health care is in critical condition. Currently there are an estimated 43 million Americans who are without health insurance. Add to that the millions more who are underinsured — those with inadequate benefits or with riders or waivers attached to their policies. One study indicates that as many as 50 percent of those who are insured are actually underinsured.

As we enter the twenty-first century, the United States remains the only industrialized country in the world (besides South Africa) without a national health insurance program. Instead we continue to rely primarily on private industry to provide a public need. And it is this approach, says insurance expert Robert Enteen, that is at the heart of our national health care problem. "In contrast to education, health insurance in this country is treated as a commodity rather than a right. After all, we guarantee free public education to every child up to a certain age. But we've yet to come to terms with how we can provide health insurance protection to all Americans."

As a result, far too many cancer survivors (as well as others with serious medical conditions) find that the current system undermines their chances for leading a healthy and happy life. According to consumer advocate Ralph Nader, the goal is clear: "We need to completely replace our present system with a fair and comprehensive program of health insurance that will cover everyone and will emphasize quality control, cost control, and preventive medicine."

National health insurance is not a new idea. Politicians have been batting it around Congress for decades. Although public opinion polls reflect that most Americans believe the financing of our health care system needs an overhaul, no one seems to know exactly how or when it will happen. Washington may eventually get around to revamping the system, but if past political battles are any indication, legislation is likely to languish until the situation reaches catastrophic proportions. Observes Ralph Nader:

ॐ If people think we can leave the health care problem to a few senators to fix, they're wrong. The best chance we have of changing the system is through consumer advocacy, and by convincing citizens that real power lies in grass roots organizations. People have to begin rallying 'round the proverbial village square. Each town needs to organize its own cooperative health clinics. If universal health insurance is going to work at all, it must emerge from local community organizations that extend all the way up to the national level. That way, by the time a universal health insurance law is passed, the program will have a solid base at the community level. ॐ

National health insurance isn't going to bring about utopia, but it just might give us the chance we need to rearrange our medical priorities.

Nevertheless, the insurance problem is likely to get worse before it gets better. That doesn't mean you should throw up your hands in despair and accept the role of victim. The seemingly insignificant act of fighting for your own decent coverage is a small yet powerful and courageous example of self-advocacy.

Such self-advocacy doesn't necessarily mean you will change the system overnight. But it will provide you a shot at getting your voice heard. And it just might give you some measure of power over your health care destiny. Says Nader:

ॐ People *can* make a difference. Look at all the cancer survivors there are! If enough of them work together, they can make things happen. After all, look what the disabled were able to do on disability rights. The media aren't interested in reporting on closed-door advocacy. They like to see people speaking up and demanding change. The question is, when are you going to start? ॐ

Resources for Insurance Information

The following agencies and associations can provide you with further information on health insurance issues.

Agency for Health Care Policy and Research (AHCPR)
Web site: info@ahcpr.gov
An agency of the Department of Health and Human Services that researches and disseminates information aimed at improving the quality of health care, reducing its cost, and broadening access to essential services. AHCPR offers a fax-on-demand service (24 hours a day, 7 days a week). To access their information, fax (301) 594-2800, then press 1.

Blue Cross/Blue Shield Associations
233 North Michigan Ave.
Chicago, IL 60601
(312) 297-6000
Web site: www.bluecares.com/feat/find.html
Provides information on Blue Cross/Blue Shield coverage offered in every state, including the availability of biannual open enrollment periods.

Champaign County Health Care Consumers Organization
44 E. Main St., Suite 208
Champaign, IL 61820
(217) 352-6533
A nonprofit community-based organization dedicated to promoting health care reform through consumer advocacy, community education, and collective action on the part of concerned citizens.

Communicating for Agriculture, Inc.
112 E. Lincoln Ave.
Fergus Falls, MN 56537
(612) 854-9005
Web site: www.caine.org
A national rural organization offering up-to-date information on high-

risk insurance pools. Since 1975, Communicating for Agriculture has served as a strong advocate for the establishment of state-run risk pools. Call (800) 432-3276 to order their annual publication, Comprehensive Health Insurance for High-Risk Individuals.

Comprehensive Omnibus Budget Reconciliation Act (COBRA)
U.S. Department of Labor
Pension and Welfare Benefits Administration
Room N-5619
200 Constitution Ave., NW
Washington, D.C.
(202) 219-8776

Employee Retirement and Income Security Act (ERISA)
U.S. Department of Labor
Pension and Welfare Benefits Administration
Room N-5619
200 Constitution Ave., NW
Washington, D.C.
(202) 219-8776

Equal Employment Opportunity Commission
Call toll-free for their Americans with Disabilities Act Information Line at (800) 669-EEOC *(voice) or* (800) 800-3302 *(TDD).*

Health Axis
Web site: www.healthaxis.com
An online source for affordable, high-quality health insurance. Health Axis can help you find and purchase the right health plan, eliminating much of the usual paperwork and high costs.

Heath Insurance Association of America
555 13th Street, NW
Washington, D.C. 20036
(202) 824-1600
Web site: www.haii.org

An industry association that represents commercial insurers,
providing information to the public on health, life, and disability
insurance.

Health Insurance Portability and Accountability Act
(HIPAA)
Health Care Financing Administration
200 Independence Ave., S W
Washington, D.C. 20201
(202) 690-6145
Web site: www.hhs.gov

HealthTracker PC
Web site: www.shareware.com
Download this free program for an easy and practical means
of storing all your medical information in one place.

Medical Information Bureau, Inc. (MIB)
P.O. Box 105
Essex Station
Boston, MA 02112
(617) 426-3660
Write to the MIB to request a copy of your medical records so that
you can verify the information and correct any inaccuracies. Call the
MIB to find out the type of information it will need to process
your request, such as your date of birth, social security number, and
so on.

Medicare and Medicaid Information

For Medicare information (eligibility, enrollment, benefits, and so on), contact your local social security office or call (800) 772-1213. Medicaid is administered through state agencies; for information, contact your local welfare or medical assistance office.

National Association of Claims Assistance Professionals
5329 S. Main St.
Suite 102
Downers Grove, IL 60515
(800) 660-0665
Call NACAP for information on private medical claims-processing companies.

National Association of Insurance Commissioners (NAIC)
Insurance companies and HMOs are licensed and regulated by the state. For information on your state's insurance department or insurance commissioner, call the NAIC at (816) 842-3600.

National Coalition for Cancer Survivorship (NCCS)
1010 Wayne Ave.
Silver Spring, MD 20910
(301) 565-9670
To order What Cancer Survivors Need to Know About Health Insurance, *call (301) 650-8868.*

National Committee for Quality Assurance
(800) 839-6487
Web site: www.ncqu.org/consumer.htm
A nonprofit organization that assesses and reports on HMO quality. Its brochure, Choosing Quality: Finding the Health Plan That's Right for You, *is available to consumers free of charge.*

The National Consumer Helpline
(800) 942-4242
Web site: www.iii.org

National Patient Advocate Foundation
780 Pilot House Dr.
Suite 100-C
Newport News, VA 23606
(757) 873-6668
Web site: www.npaf.org

Underwriters Laboratories
333 Pfingsten Rd.
Northbrook, IL 60062
(847) 272-8800
Publishes the annual guide Who Writes What in Life and Health Insurance.

7

When the Résumé Includes Cancer

IN WESTERN SOCIETY, what you do for a living is a vital measure of who you are. Work is your public voice, a cultural ID tag. It is also an important source of security, self-esteem, and, if you're lucky, happiness. Whether you toil for love or money, power or prestige, work provides you with the chance to fulfill your ambitions and fix a course in life.

For cancer survivors, employment takes on added significance: going back to work means getting back to normal. But for some, the transition back is not always smooth sailing. A sense of personal vulnerability may be compounded by prejudicial attitudes and hardcore economic policies. Workplace discrimination might be blatant and overt, such as outright dismissal, reduced company benefits, an unwanted transfer, or rejection of a job application. More often, though, it takes a subtler form. You may notice it in the hesitancy before a handshake, in the glances and whispers of coworkers, or in the promotions or pay hikes that never quite materialize.

Nancy Davenport-Ennis, the founder and executive director of the National Patient Advocate Foundation, states:

& prolem Most of the cancer survivors who call our office with job discrimination problems today tend to be employees in management positions. For many of them, the discriminatory problem boils down to financial issues having to do with the company's group health insurance. If an employee is diagnosed with cancer, that will probably trigger a rate increase in premiums for all employees. So the way the employer sees it, the way to control the overhead on health insurance is to limit the number of employees with chronic or debilitating health problems.

The fear of discrimination itself can be enough to diminish job opportunities. For instance, many survivors remain in undesirable jobs or careers because they worry that their cancer history might hinder their chances of being hired elsewhere. Some are even reluctant to take advantage of sick leave, fearing that they may jeopardize their jobs by doing so.

Employment discrimination can be especially difficult for young survivors who have little or no previous experience in the job market. Many find it is an uphill battle convincing potential employers that a cancer history is not an impediment to a productive career.

This was Tim's experience when he applied in 1983 for a job with his hometown police department. Tim, forty, was treated for Hodgkin's disease when he was eleven years old. His boyhood ambition of becoming a law enforcement official, perhaps even an FBI agent, remained undaunted by his bout with cancer. Eight years later, and a week before beginning his law school entrance exams, he enrolled in the police force.

There was one hitch, however. After he applied for the job, Tim had to contend with a city policy governing the hiring of cancer survivors.

  At the time I took the preliminary police department test, no one informed me that I might be rejected because of a history of cancer. I'd already completed one year of law school when I was finally notified by the Nassau County Police Department to report for further testing. The background check involved a medical history and exam. I filled out the forms and then took the physical. On the form, there was a checklist that included "malignant tumor —

history or presence of." Since I didn't see any point in lying about it, I checked the box.

After reviewing my application, the civil service commission doctors said that my cancer history disqualified me. We argued, and they finally suggested I go on and take the psychological profile exam. I did, and I passed. But they disqualified me anyway. It seemed unbelievable to me that the civil service commission, whose job it is to prohibit discrimination in the public sector, was basically promulgating a blatant discriminatory policy of its own.

Outraged, I contacted the civil liberties union and the attorney general's office, and together we threatened the police department with a lawsuit. Just before we went to court, they turned around and reversed their ruling, reappointing me to the list of eligible candidates.

In the end they backed down. However, I then learned that although they had reappointed me to the list, they weren't going to change their policies, and so I changed my mind about joining the force. Instead, I teamed up with a local senator. Together we drafted legislation that would prohibit the New York Civil Service Department from discriminating against cancer survivors. The bill easily sailed through both congressional houses in New York, but was vetoed by the governor several times, until 1992, when it finally passed into law. &

Now an attorney in private practice, Tim continues to lecture and advocate on behalf of the workplace rights of cancer survivors.

The Myths Behind Workplace Cancer-Based Discrimination

Tim's case poses the question that all survivors ask: If my medical team considers me fit to work, why shouldn't potential employers? The answer is clear: the medical community's view of cancer is based on a full understanding of the disease and greater optimism about treatment efficacy. Popular attitudes, however, remain tinged with fear and stereotypic thinking. For centuries, myths and mis-understandings surrounding cancer have served as the wellspring for prejudice and discrimination. As recently as the 1950s, cancerphobia continued to be so deeply rooted in Western culture that doctors frequently withheld telling cancer patients the exact nature of their diagnosis.

Social attitudes and legislation that serves to sway them have cer-tainly evolved since then. In today's world, most employers treat those with a cancer history with fairness and compassion. Nonethe-less, old ways of thinking die hard. Despite the progress made in diagnosis and treatment, cancer's reputation remains moored to an assortment of punishing myths. Three in particular continue to in-fluence the way some employers and coworkers perceive survivors.

The "Death Sentence" Myth

This myth assumes that cancer is an inevitably fatal disease, and that those who have it aren't destined to live long. Employers who buy into this way of thinking are reluctant to hire a cancer survivor.

Ignorance fuels this myth. People are often surprised to learn that cancer accounts for just 20 percent of deaths in the United States, whereas cardiovascular disease kills twice as many people. In fact, cancer is now considered one of *the most curable* of chronic diseases. The National Cancer Institute reports that more than half of those diagnosed with cancer today will survive their illness and go on to lead full, productive lives. The current long-term survival rate has increased significantly from forty years ago, when the figure hovered around 30 percent. Survival rates for many childhood and adolescent cancers are particularly impressive, with rates as high as 90 percent.

The "Unproductive Worker" Myth

An employer may worry that an employee recovering from can-cer won't be able to perform adequately on the job or may require assistance from coworkers. Some employers also suspect that turnover and absentee rates will be higher for those with a cancer history.

This myth was dispelled years ago by two landmark studies. The first of these was conducted by the Metropolitan Life Insurance Company. From 1959 to 1972, Metropolitan tracked the employment records of seventy-four survivors and found no difference in absenteeism, turnover, or work performance from those of nonsurvivor employees. According to their findings, not one survivor had been dismissed as a result of poor performance. The results were so encouraging that the study concluded that the hiring of cancer survivors was "sound industrial practice."

In 1972, a study by the American Telephone and Telegraph Company revealed that approximately 80 percent of 1,351 AT&T employees diagnosed with cancer returned to their jobs after completion of treatment. The study concluded that a cancer diagnosis did not automatically shorten or subvert an employee's productive life.

The "Cancer Is Contagious" Myth

The persistence of this myth is testament to how deeply ingrained cancerphobia remains in our culture. Cancer is no more contagious than arthritis or poor vision. Still, some people act as though it is, in effect socially quarantining the survivor.

Unbelievable as it sounds, I once heard from a survivor who was fired from his job as a restaurant chef because it was feared he might contaminate the food. A woman I know was asked during a job interview if she had ever been seriously ill. When she answered that she was a survivor of childhood leukemia, her interviewer asked, "How did you catch that?"

Some people cling to cancer mythology the way others entertain superstitious or "magical" thinking. They may have heard cancer isn't contagious, but they aren't taking any chances.

Your Workplace Rights Under the Law

Whether you have a job or are looking for one, keep in mind that discrimination based on a history of cancer is a violation of federal law, and may also be in violation of state law. An employer is legally bound to treat an employee (or potential employee) with a history of cancer no differently from any other employee, provided he or she qualifies for the job and is proficient at performing the tasks and responsibilities involved. A clear understanding of your legal rights can foster the self-confidence and sense of self-advocacy you need to stand up to discriminatory practices.

Federal Laws

The Americans with Disabilities Act of 1990 (ADA). Arguably the most significant disability rights legislation in decades, the ADA was originally intended to prohibit discrimination against individuals with a perceived disability or history of a disability. Those instrumental in passing the ADA maintained that it would offer significant protection to millions of Americans who have medical conditions or impairments (such as cancer, AIDS, epilepsy, diabetes) that might leave them vulnerable to job discrimination. However, a recent Supreme Court decision sharply narrowed the scope of this federal antidiscrimination law. Ruling on a key aspect of the ADA, the Court put forth a more restrictive view of the ADA's definition of disability, by determining that protection did not extend to those with disabilities or impairments that can be controlled or corrected by medication or other devices. In other words, individuals with *remediable conditions* are not, under the law, considered disabled.

"Where this leaves the ADA is with a huge gaping hole right at its heart," observed Professor Chai Feldblum of Georgetown Law School, one of the drafters of the law. The decision, he added, "creates the absurd result of a person being disabled enough to be fired from a job, but not disabled enough to challenge the firing."

While this recent ruling has in effect diluted the original intent of the ADA, survivors should still be aware of the law's key provisions. For instance, the ADA extends to companies in the private sector with fifteen or more employees and covers all employment practices, including job applications and hiring, advancement and compensation, layoffs and firings, leaves of absence, and fringe benefits.

This wide-ranging civil rights bill makes it illegal for an employer to discriminate against a qualified applicant or employee who is disabled, has a history of a disability, or is perceived as having a disability. In this regard, the ADA protects cancer survivors from discrimination based on their medical histories. It also forbids discrimination against disabled people in all public services (such as state and local government offices), public accommodations (hotels, restaurants, shopping centers, and so on), transportation, and telecommunication.

The ADA states that employers must provide "reasonable accommodation" to qualified disabled employees. (Reasonable accommodation denotes any assistance — for instance, more flexible hours — that a disabled employee may need to facilitate work duties.) Originally, the law contained the same broad definition of "disability" put forth in Section 504 of the Federal Rehabilitation Act of 1973, although as mentioned above, that definition, as it pertains to the ADA, was recently pared back. You can learn more about reasonable job accommodation under the ADA by contacting the Job Accommodation Network at (800) 526-7234.

Employers are also prohibited from asking medical questions before offering applicants a job unless their health history has strict bearing on work performance. Nor can applicants be required to undergo a preemployment medical exam unless it is (1) job-related, and (2) requested of all employees. The ADA also permits medical leave in addition to that offered under the Family and Medical Leave Act, although no employee can assume that an employer will hold open any job indefinitely.

Under the ADA, survivors may seek remedies against employers who violate the law, including injunctive relief (to halt the discriminatory practice) and back pay, if they are denied a job or fired as a result of their disability. (Note, however, that the law applies only to those companies with fifteen or more employees; those working for businesses with fewer than fifteen employees will have to look to state laws for protection.) The Americans with Disabilities Act is enforced by the U.S. Equal Employment Opportunity Commission (EEOC). Survivors who believe they are victims of workplace discrimination should immediately contact their nearest EEOC office at (800) 669-4000 for information about procedures and deadlines for filing a complaint. Do so promptly, however; a delay could invalidate your claim.

The Rehabilitation Act of 1973. Prior to the Americans with Disabilities Act, the Rehabilitation Act was a survivor's best option for a legal remedy against work-related discrimination. Because this law extends only to a limited number of employers, however, it fell short of offering protection to all survivors.

The Rehabilitation Act, amended in 1978 and 1984, prohibits discrimination against the disabled by employers who receive federal funding or federal contracts of more than $2,500 annually. The law also protects federal employees. Section 504 of the act protects against discrimination in all federally assisted programs and activities, including hospitals, schools, and colleges.

Section 7(7) of the act defines a "handicapped individual" as "any person who (i) has a physical or mental impairment which substantially limits one or more of such person's major life activities, (ii) has a record of such an impairment, or (iii) is regarded as having such an impairment." This broad definition includes people who may not consider themselves handicapped or disabled, including many cancer survivors. Although the act does not specifically list cancer as a disability, the U.S. Supreme Court has determined that cancer is covered under this law.

The Rehabilitation Act prohibits covered employers from discrimination in hiring, promotions, transfers, wages and salaries, benefits (including health and life insurance), and termination. In addition, a covered employer cannot require an applicant to undergo a medical or physical examination prior to offering that person a job. Once an applicant has been offered a job, however, a medical history or exam may be required, but only if it is required of other applicants. Under this law, employers are required to provide "reasonable accommodation" to disabled employees (this is discussed in greater detail later in the chapter).

Survivors who take legal action under Sections 501 and 504 of the act can file for job reinstatement, attorneys' fees, injunctive relief, and back pay. Employers who violate the law risk having their federal funds withheld, including cancelation of any federal contracts. Sections 503 and 504 of the Rehabilitation Act of 1973 are handled by separate government offices (see the listings at the end of this chapter).

If you choose to file a complaint under the Rehabilitation Act, contact the Equal Employment Opportunity Commission at (800) 669-4000. The EEOC routinely performs "legal triage" for those persons seeking information about how best to handle employment discrimination problems.

The Family and Medical Leave Act. Under this federal law, employers with fifty or more employees are required to provide up to twelve weeks per year of unpaid, job-protected leave to any employee in need of time off to attend to a personal serious illness or that of a spouse, child, or parent. In addition, the law also covers employees who must, for "medically necessary" reasons, reduce or reshuffle their work schedules. (Employers do have the right to request a note from the employee's doctor, certifying the medical reason for the leave.) Under the Family and Medical Leave Act, an employee's health benefits are protected, and at the end of the allotted leave the employee is guaranteed a return to the same position or its equivalent. To be eligible, an employee must have worked at least twenty-five hours a week for a minimum of one year.

Complaints regarding the Family and Medical Leave Act must be filed with the Employment Standards Administration, Wage and Hour Division of the U.S. Department of Labor.

State Laws

In addition to these federal statutes, most states have laws proscribing employment discrimination in both the private and public sector against people with disabilities. The amount and type of protection available vary from state to state. Several states — California, Vermont, and Florida, to name a few — and the District of Columbia, have laws that expressly prohibit discrimination based on a cancer history. The California Fair Employment and Housing Act (FEHA), for instance, prohibits employment discrimination based on a "medical condition" or "physical handicap." The "medical condition" defined in FEHA refers to "any health impairment related to or associated with a diagnosis of cancer, for which a person has been rehabilitated or cured, based on competent medical evidence." The law covers all California businesses employing five or more people.

To learn about your state laws, contact the state agency that enforces employment rights, your local bar association or civil service commission, or cancer support groups that offer employment-related resources. They can explain the methods for filing a complaint and the filing deadlines.

How to Address Workplace Discrimination

Now that you have an understanding of the myths that can provoke employment discrimination as well as the laws that prohibit it, you should be aware of how both can affect your entry or return to the workforce. Your own attitude and behavior also play an important part in how well you finesse an encounter with cancer-based discrimination.

To Tell or Not to Tell: Job Applications and Interviews

Job interviews are by their very nature stressful occasions. You will feel particular pressure if you are worrying about your health history. Even with an enlightened employer, it is not easy to explain cancer-related gaps on your résumé. There you are, diligently filling out an application when there appears the question asking whether you've had cancer. Your pen hovers over the boxes marked yes and no. Which one will you check?

First of all, the question itself is illegal. Under the Americans with Disabilities Act, employers may not inquire about (or request records of) your medical history or require you to take a medical examination prior to offering you a job (unless the exam is required of all other applicants in your particular job category). Employee health examinations are only allowed when they are strictly job related and consistent with business necessity (that is, to determine an appropriate accommodation for a disability).

Disability rights advocates are divided over how to handle the issue of disclosure. Cancer survivor advocate and disability rights lawyer Barbara Hoffman recommends that survivors not volunteer any cancer-related information unless your medical condition is directly job-related and affects your ability to do the work. "There's always a risk when you disclose information that it will be used against you," says Hoffman. "It's a personal choice, and ultimately you should be comfortable with your decision."

Attorney Tim Calonita, whose fight against employment discrimination was recounted earlier in this chapter, advises the opposite approach:

ॐ Use your cancer history as a sword, not a shield, and in the process do a little saber-rattling. I counsel survivors to tell a potential employer: "Listen, I've fought cancer. I've handled chemotherapy. I can take on anything this job throws at me." Be proactive. Set the stage. Put a positive, prideful spin on it. You'd be amazed at how empowering and effective this approach can be. ॐ

Ultimately, any decision you make on disclosure should be based on personal style and what feels right to you. I myself chose for many years to avoid the issue; unless I was asked directly, I never mentioned my medical history. But I suppose growing older has made me bolder. A few years ago, I decided to test the waters, as it were, and applied for several job openings that appealed to me. Filling out an application, my eyes fell on the question regarding a history of serious illnesses. I left it blank. During the interview, I was asked why by the personnel director. "Since the question is illegal, I didn't see the point," I replied. The personnel director admitted that the application form needed updating and went on to recommend me for the job, which I subsequently declined. On to the next job interview, this one for a position as regional fashion manager for a department store. The subject came up, and I was both candid and passionate in relating what I'd gained from my experience with cancer. The interviewer later informed me that it was my forthright, strong-willed style that assured me the job if I wanted it.

However you decided to handle the question if and when it arises, remember one important bit of advice: *Don't lie.* If you lie on a job or insurance application, and are later found out, the revelation can serve as grounds for dismissal (or in the case of insurance, cancelation of your policy).

Even though there are laws in place, don't expect discriminatory hiring practices to vanish anytime soon. As health care costs and insurance premiums maintain their upward spiral, employers will continue to find and utilize loopholes in the law. It is over this bottom-line issue that your interests and those of an employer are most likely to be at cross-purposes. This is a particular problem for smaller businesses, which, unlike large corporations, don't have a large pool of employees or the budget to absorb higher insurance rates. As a result, many smaller firms are forced to choose between affordable insurance coverage and the welfare of an employee with a cancer history.

Of growing concern too is the controversial issue of genetic testing in the workplace — its use and abuse as a screening tool by employers. Several recent state-level court cases concerning an employer's use of genetic information highlight the dramatic and possibly ominous consequences this issue could have on all our lives. A simple, seemingly innocuous blood test during a preemployment medical exam will possibly reveal predispositions you have to one or more serious medical conditions. In such cases, ethical issues of privacy and confidentiality collide head-on with an employer's desire to monitor workers for drug abuse or to screen out those who may contribute to rising health care costs. As it now stands, states with laws governing genetic antidiscrimination also extend to health insurance application processes. The Equal Employment Opportunity Commission, however, has determined that genetic testing falls under the ADA, so survivors who are discriminated against by their employer or employer-based health plan solely because of genetic testing can file with the EEOC. (For an update on laws, contact the Council for Responsible Genetics: 617-868-0870.) Think of it as genetic destiny perhaps, but until federal legislation outlaws such discrimination, consider it a real possibility that your DNA will be used against you.

Additional Suggestions for Job Interviews

- *Don't disqualify yourself.* According to attorney Tim Calonita, "Sometimes the problem lies with the survivors' attitude; how they perceive and project themselves. In effect, they discriminate against themselves, automatically assuming they can't hold certain jobs. They use their cancer as scapegoat, as an excuse to take themselves out of the running."

- *Stress your ability to do the job.* Should you have any visible disability secondary to your cancer, find an opportunity during the interview to discuss it with the employer, offering assurance that it in no way prevents you from doing the job. This will also give you a chance to alleviate the employer's fears and answer questions regarding any possible on-the-job accommodations that your disability may require. Keep in mind that it is the employer's obligation to make it possible for a qualified person with a disability to do the job, no matter when the disability was made known.

An employer should be interested in only one issue: can you do the job? Your role during a job interview is that of salesperson. What you are selling is your ability to help the employer run the business as effectively as possible, so conduct the interview on those terms. Be positive and assertive. Impress upon the employer your capabilities and strengths. Don't hesitate to say at the end of the interview, "I want this job, and this is how I intend to carry out the responsibilities involved." As survivor advocate Barbara Hoffman says, "You have no moral or legal obligation to talk about your cancer unless it has some bearing on job performance. After all, you're looking for a job, not approval."

An equally important point: try not to appear overly concerned about the type of insurance coverage or benefits package offered. Your potential boss wants you to be first and foremost interested in the job. Once you've been officially offered the position, then by all means look into benefits.

- *Get your doctor's endorsement.* An employee's physical limitations are obviously going to be a concern to any employer. If a potential employer has questions or doubts about your ability to perform the job, ask your employer to contact your doctor. (Or better yet, be prepared, and bring a letter from your doctor with you to the interview.) Everyone likes to be reassured by experts, and a call or letter from your physician will give your application a medical "seal of approval." Many survivors have found this strategy to be highly effective.

- *In specific situations, physical examinations are a condition of hiring.* A medical history or physical exam may be considered an essential part of determining whether a person is appropriate for a particular job. In Tim's case, law enforcement departments called for all applicants to be screened for any medical conditions or impairments that could create on-the-job problems. If physical fitness is a requirement for the position — as it would be for any job where the public's health and safety are at stake — then medical screening would be appropriate.

• *Don't give in to discrimination.* If, during or after a job interview, you suspect that an employer has engaged in discriminatory practices, you have the right to take action. You can do this first by letting your interviewer know, in a calm and diplomatic way, that you are aware of the laws protecting cancer survivors. Then bring it to the employer's attention that you intend to pursue the matter further.

Discriminatory Practices in the Workplace

Employment discrimination is by no means limited to hiring practices. More often it happens on the job, where the overt or covert prejudicial attitudes of employers and coworkers can result in biased behavior. According to Nancy Davenport-Ennis of the National Patient Advocate Foundation, there are several workplace scenarios that may constitute discriminatory behavior on the part of employers:

1. A "work slowdown" scenario involves cancer survivors returning to work only to find that their hours or job duties have been cut, in effect demoting them to the status of part-time employee. In the process, health benefits may be cut or eliminated.

2. In the "overtime" scenario, an employer suggests to a returning employee that he or she needs to make up the work time lost due to treatment. Many survivors, feeling responsible and perhaps guilty, will acquiesce to this enforced work overload. Before long, the survivor may be working sixty or more hours a week, a schedule that would physically tax anyone, let alone someone recovering from a major illness. At some point, the employer, feigning concern, will then ask the employee, "Are you able to maintain the projects we've assigned to you? We are a little worried that there may have been a slowdown in your performance and are concerned you may not get these projects in on time."

The employee, feeling pressured, may request a transfer to another department. The trap becomes all too visible when the employee discovers that there are no transfers available, or, if there are, the transfer will entail a reduction in benefits.

3. The "transfer" scenario has management informing the returning survivor of his or her relocation to another position, a different level of management, or even a move to an office in another city. The inconvenience of such a transfer often results in the desired effect: resignation.

Of course, this is not to imply that every transfer, demotion, or other career curve balls necessarily involve discriminatory attitudes or behavior. Many other factors can come into play, such as office politics, seniority, your own work performance and attitude, even the state of the economy.

But let's assume that you are performing your job satisfactorily and you are still passed over for that long-awaited promotion. How can you determine whether or not the action is discriminatory?

Begin by taking a hard look at the situation. Try to understand exactly what has happened. Can you say with absolute certainty that cancer played a part in it? Some survivors are quick to interpret denial of a promotion, a demotion, or an undesirable transfer as evidence of cancer-based discrimination. They allow themselves to fall into the "victim" trap, where every slight is perceived to be a sure sign of prejudice.

It's easy to misinterpret a ruthless yet legitimate business decision as a discriminatory action, especially if that decision is contrary to your wishes or expectations. Try to depersonalize the situation and determine what else might have influenced it.

By all means, don't rule out your own attitude and orientation toward work. It could be that cancer has altered your priorities, and the driving ambition you once had for work has now shifted to other means of self-fulfillment. Such a change could in itself greatly influence the speed and direction of your career.

It's also possible that cancer has had a deleterious effect on your self-esteem. You may no longer feel capable of competing with "healthy" coworkers. Self-doubt is more detrimental than any physical disability or discriminatory action. In short, confidence is contagious. If you have faith in your abilities, chances are others will too.

If, however, after weighing the situation, you are convinced that discriminatory behavior exists, take action. The information provided below is not intended as legal advice, but rather as suggestions on how you might resolve a perceived discriminatory action.

- *Gather information.* Before attempting to resolve your grievance, you may want to consult with an employment rights agency or cancer advocacy group in your community. These organizations can help you sort out your legal rights and refer you to other resources.

- *Determine how you want to handle your situation.* You may want to work through your problem internally, either by dealing directly with your supervisor, personnel director, or union representative or by taking advantage of whatever administrative complaint procedure your company offers employees. If not, you may find it necessary to file a formal complaint with an administrative agency outside the company. Try to determine what would be the most effective and least frustrating way to resolve the situation.

- *Document your claim.* Be sure to keep a record of any action you perceive to be discriminatory. This written record will be helpful later on if you decide to take legal action. Include details of the incident such as the date, the time, and the names of people involved, including any coworkers who happen to have witnessed it.

- *Research your rights under the law.* Familiarize yourself with both state and federal laws protecting the on-the-job rights of the disabled. Find out where you stand and if your problem can be defined as discriminatory. Be aware that many disability laws require that you contact specific administrative agencies before you take legal action. Also, determine what the deadlines are for applying. If you overlook or in some way fail to comply with these administrative procedures, your claim could be invalidated.

* *Find a lawyer.* If you have the funds and fortitude, you may choose to retain a lawyer, preferably one who specializes in disability rights or employment law. If you can't afford to hire an attorney, contact a survivor advocacy organization or your local bar association. They may be able to refer you to a legal aid lawyer at little or no cost.

However you choose to handle your situation, you have a right not to be discriminated against because of your cancer history. A caveat: one of the reasons on-the-job discrimination can be so difficult to identify is that an employer's prejudicial attitudes are often cloaked in concern and solicitude. My own experience revealed just how subtle this kind of discrimination can be. In the first chapter of this book, I described how I was once up for promotion with a large cosmetics firm. I lost out when a coworker suggested to the company's vice president that my cancer history might interfere with my ability to do the job. It was later explained to me that I had been "spared" the promotion because it was thought I might find the extensive travel required too strenuous.

Few things are as distressing as someone deciding the fate of your career for you. It's even more infuriating when your employer does it "for your own good." No one has the right to prevent you from fulfilling your ambitions and enacting career decisions. Of course, you must know your limitations and what you can realistically achieve. But don't shy away from fighting back if office prejudice is interfering with your ambitions.

Office Ostracism

One workplace worry that plagues survivors is determining how to deal with the insensitive or inappropriate responses of coworkers. Although the public is far less cancerphobic than it once was, I still hear from survivors who were shunned at work or subject to hostile remarks. A somewhat bizarre example of such discrimination is the experience of a survivor named Veronica, forty-four, who took time off from her job as an administrative assistant at a manufacturing firm to undergo treatment for early stage cervical cancer. Her first day back at work was, as she describes it, a rather "sticky" affair:

ॐ Three weeks after my operation, I headed right back to work. The morning of my return I found a big bouquet of flowers sitting on my desk. Everyone at the office was terrific, very friendly and solicitous. As a "welcome back" gesture, several coworkers announced that they wanted to treat me to lunch. I was beginning to feel like queen for a day.

As it turned out, not everyone was thrilled to have me back. After I returned from lunch, I grabbed a cup of coffee and returned to my desk. Right away I noticed something was wrong; the desk was damp and slightly sticky. It also smelled funny. I picked up the phone and noticed that it was sticky too. So were the files, my pens and pencils, the computer — everything on and around my desk had a slight film of *something* on it.

I immediately asked my boss about it. At first she thought I was joking, but once she sat down at my desk she was as baffled as I was. I asked around and no one would give me a satisfactory answer. I decided to check with Tom, a friend and coworker. He looked so sheepish, I could tell right away that he knew something. I badgered him a bit and he finally told me that a couple of the secretaries sitting near me had decided to disinfect my entire office with Lysol, just in case what I had was catching. ॐ

Veronica asked her supervisor for suggestions on how to handle the situation. They decided to organize an informal "cancer conference." The following morning, a memo was issued to all office personnel. Everyone was asked to meet in the conference room.

Veronica supplied the facts, talking about her recent illness as she handed out pamphlets on cervical cancer:

&⅋ I filled them in on the details, making it very clear that cancer was in no way a communicable disease. I didn't name names, and I didn't get angry. I simply stated that I thought they might have questions about what had happened to me, and that this was the best way to handle it. I told them that except for the loss of my uterus, I was the same old Veronica.

Even though most of my coworkers were already fairly knowledgeable about cancer, I could tell that the discussion made an impact, and not just on the Lysol squad. I think it put everyone at ease to hear me talk openly about my experience and see the information in black and white. The meeting gave everyone a chance to answer all the unspoken questions they'd been too embarrassed or afraid to ask. It wasn't exactly the easiest thing I've ever done, but the results were worth it. &⅋

No one wants to be on the receiving end of office gossip or discriminatory behavior. And nobody should be expected to accept it. Instead, combat it through information and education. Should you encounter office prejudice, consider the following:

- *Examine your own attitude as objectively as possible.* Are your coworkers treating you differently since you've returned, or are they merely reacting to the signals you're sending? Survivors often have mixed feelings about what they want out of life after cancer. Look inside yourself before you misinterpret the actions and attitudes of others. Consider whether or not the problem is due to your own difficulty in readjusting to the workplace.

- *Talk to the boss.* It is the responsibility of your boss or office supervisor to ensure that the office runs smoothly and the environment promotes productivity. If a coworker's prejudicial actions are interfering with your ability to get the job done, ask your boss to act as intermediary.

- *Organize an office meeting.* This approach worked for Veronica, as it has for several other Cancervive members. (Of course, confirm it with your boss or supervisor first.) Also, consider distributing pamphlets or articles that describe the kind of cancer you had. Both the American Cancer Society and the National Cancer Institute publish materials that clearly explain the facts about specific types of cancers. If you can arrange it, invite a social worker or nurse from your hospital to speak to the group.

You may discover, as Veronica did, that the easiest way to squelch office fear and prejudice is to be as candid as possible about your cancer experience. Of course, that doesn't mean you need to bare your soul and reveal highly personal details. Instead, emphasize the positive. For the one or two individuals in your office who may still cling stubbornly to the myths about cancer, a clear insight into your illness might be just the thing to change their minds.

If your illness has resulted in physical impairments, fellow employees will no doubt be uncertain of how to respond to you. Take the initiative and break the ice, and don't forget the power of laughter. After all, one of the easiest ways to disarm people is to make them laugh. If you can accept your disability, even laugh about it, why shouldn't your coworkers? Veronica offers an example of how a sense of humor can diffuse tension. "One of the men in my office didn't know what to say to me. He seemed so uptight and embarrassed. Then one day I mentioned to him that thanks to my hysterectomy, I was saving a bundle on contraceptives. We both had a good laugh, and now he's not half as nervous around me as he used to be."

- *Consider filing a formal complaint.* As a last resort, you may want to consider taking legal action — but only as a last resort. It is very difficult to prove office harassment. Also, a lawsuit may cause you to lose your job and/or your friendships with coworkers. Notes survivor advocate Barbara Hoffman:

& We all tend to forget that there's no law out there that says people can't be jerks. A coworker's action has to be fairly blatant before you should even consider talking to a lawyer. By blatant, I mean any action or behavior that impedes your ability to get the job done. In most instances, diplomacy and goodwill work a lot better than formal complaints and lawsuits. However, if after trying all other options, a coworker is continuing to make your work life impossible, this may be the only way to resolve it. &⁸

Vocational Rehabilitation

Although most survivors are physically able to return to work, some find that their cancer has caused permanent changes or restrictions that limit their former capabilities. If either a physical or a mental impairment has made it difficult for you to return to your job, consider redirecting your talents and skills through job retraining. Help is available through your state-run Vocational Rehabilitation Administration.

Recovering cancer patients often assume that vocational rehabilitation is limited to people with obvious impairments, such as amputees or persons who have had laryngectomies. It isn't. Cancer treatment can also result in impairments, such as loss of hearing, agility, or strength, which can directly affect your ability to resume your former line of work. Others undergo subtler, less perceptible changes. Survivors of brain cancer, for example, often have no outward signs of impairment yet may struggle with memory loss, motor skill problems, and cognitive functioning. Total rehabilitation — physical, psychosocial, and vocational — is essential to every cancer patient's recovery. Regardless of your disability, the objective is to get your life and career goals back on track.

Fritz is a survivor who took advantage of a rehabilitation program to redirect his career after cancer. The twenty-eight-year-old aspiring journalist recently described how he was fired from his job after a bout with soft-tissue cancer.

&⁸ I developed a tumor in my abdominal cavity two years ago. At the time, I was working at a supermarket, stocking shelves at night. When I told my supervisor about the diagnosis, he suggested that I take a leave of absence until I was finished with treatment. My cancer was stage three and so I got the whole nine yards: surgery, chemo, and radiation. I needed every day of my six-month medical leave to get through it.

Two days after I returned to work, I knew I still wasn't up to par. I discovered that I could no longer do the heavy lifting that the job required. During surgery the doctors had removed some of my abdominal muscles, which made lifting heavy objects nearly impossible. That caused problems at work, since my employer required all employees to perform every store duty, from manning the cash register to stocking shelves.

My supervisor noticed the difficulty I was having and suggested I take more time off to recuperate. But I didn't want that. I was eager to work; it gave me the feeling that I was back in control of my life. I asked if I could be assigned to another position, something that wouldn't require a lot of lifting. That wasn't possible according to my supervisor; to do so would mean bumping another employee out of his position. So instead, I was laid off.

They told me I was let go because I could no longer perform the job I was hired to do. But I think they just didn't want the bother of retraining me; it was easier to replace me. I also heard through the grapevine that my supervisor was worried I might injure myself on the job or get sick again.

I think it was definitely a discriminatory move, but at that point I knew I'd have a tough time proving it. Still, I was both able and eager to work for the company in some other capacity. I had lots of experience working for other grocery stores, doing everything from checking to management. But they insisted on hanging me up on store "policy." That really upset me, because I know that several of the little old ladies working cashier have never been asked to stock shelves.

In a way, though, it all turned out for the best. I have a college degree in communications, and I'd been wanting to get into a more challenging career. This gave me the shove I needed. During one of my checkups, my doctor suggested I look into vocational rehabilitation. For the last six months I've been training with a local VR program with a view toward a career in journalism. ॐ

Most survivors have no difficulty returning to their jobs, and some find that their employers are supportive of their needs as recovering patients. As Fritz's story illustrates, however, survivors with minimum dysfunction can encounter problems if their employers are unwilling or unable to accommodate them. You may have experienced a similar situation. You want to work, but now that your old job is no longer appropriate for you, your employer isn't sure what to do. You suggest retraining. Your boss suggests you look for another job. What are your options?

The first strategy you should pursue is to determine your job rights. Under the law your employer must provide you with "reasonable accommodation," which means that the company must take steps to accommodate a disabled person's special needs. Reasonable accommodation might include modifying a work environment (for instance, to accommodate an employee's wheelchair), restructuring the job, modifying work schedules, reassigning duties, or installing special devices (such as telephones for the hearing-impaired).

But there is a catch: employers are not required to provide accommodation if they can demonstrate that it would result in "undue hardship." Attorney Barbara Hoffman points out that the definition of what constitutes undue hardship includes consideration of several factors, such as the size of the business, the cost and nature of the accommodation in question, and the number of employees who would be affected by the accommodation.

&? It depends on the particulars of each case. In a large corporation, for example, it might not be a hardship to relocate or retrain a disabled employee, even if it means shuffling around the work schedules of several coworkers. However, this could very well create a lot of disruption for a small business and therefore be considered an undue burden. In short, if your employer can prove that to retrain you or accommodate you in some other capacity would be too burdensome for the company, you could be out of luck, and out of a job. &?

There are other options. Before you go any further, however, you must acknowledge your disability and accept that it has resulted in a vocational handicap. That may sound all too obvious, but the reality is that many survivors subject themselves to the pain of repeated job rejection simply because they are reluctant to admit their handicap. They've allowed denial to interfere with their rehabilitation.

Then again, some survivors paint themselves into a different corner. They have allowed their disability to dominate their lives. These survivors often conclude that they are no longer productive because of their disability, and therefore their work life is over.

If this is your situation, it's very possible that your self-esteem and self-image are in need of rehabilitation as well. By all means, don't overlook this aspect of "retraining" yourself for the workplace through either private or group therapy. Take stock of your vocational skills and career goals. Even if cancer has severely impaired your former work abilities, remember that you still have much to offer the world. Ask yourself how you might transform your disability into an asset. As a survivor, you bring to any job a unique store of experience, strength, and understanding that most other people lack. But it is up to you to tap into this special reserve and then promote it.

You may find it helpful to discuss your needs with a professional. An occupational therapist can provide vocational guidance and help you decide on the kind of work you want to pursue as well as the programs that can best prepare you for a new job or career. Financial support during your rehabilitation is also an important concern and should be discussed with family members.

If you feel that you would benefit from vocational rehabilitation, your doctor or a hospital social worker can refer you to a local vocational rehabilitation or community service office. You don't need a doctor's recommendation. Take the initiative and find out what you need to know about qualifying for local rehabilitation programs. To be eligible, it is generally required that you have both the capability and desire to return to the workforce. Any disability that interferes

with your normal line of work can qualify you for vocational rehabilitation assistance in the form of counseling, job training, financial
assistance, or training in the use of special equipment. Vocational rehabilitation also provides special programs such as speech lessons for
laryngectomy patients.

Every state is mandated to offer vocational rehabilitation programs. Specific qualifications vary from state to state, although survivors who qualify for social security disability automatically qualify
for such programs. Call your state rehabilitation department (listed
in the state government section of your phone directory) for further
information about requirements.

The Work Ahead: Advocacy and Consensus Building

> Never doubt that a small group of concerned, committed citizens can
> change the world. Indeed, it is the only thing that ever has.
>
> — Margaret Mead

For survivors who have encountered employment discrimination, it
is one of the most frustrating and infuriating obstacles to life after
cancer. Tim says he remains angry over the issue of cancer-based
discrimination despite his victory over the police department's hiring policy.

… There are really two battles you wage when you get cancer. First
you fight the disease. Then you may have to contend with the biased
attitudes and fears of employers and coworkers. I'm not saying
that survivors should get preferential treatment. But I do think we
should have the same chance as everyone else. And that's why I
fought back. …

For survivors like Tim, fighting back sometimes means a trip to
court. For others, like Veronica, it means fighting back one-on-one
with education, information, and a sense of humor.

My own encounter with job discrimination would have undoubtedly fared better if I had been more aware at the time of the legal remedies available to me. Since then I've learned the importance of advocacy. Had I known then what I know now, I most certainly would have fought for my employment rights. Instead I decided to start my own nonprofit organization. Now, I often joke to people, no one can fire me.

Happily, since I began Cancervive, I've noticed a perceptible change in the public's attitude regarding cancer. Although much still needs to be done, education and advocacy are slowly chipping away at the myths and misinformation. Organizations like the Employment Law Center, the National Patient Advocate Foundation, the National Coalition for Cancer Survivorship, and Cancervive continue to advance the rights of patients and survivors.

But perhaps the most significant influence on public perception can be found in the growing ranks of survivors. Scores of prominent personalities — actors, politicians, sports figures — are beating the disease and demonstrating in full light of the media that a cancer history is not incompatible with a vital, productive career. Employers need only to remember that the highest office in the land was at one time held by a cancer survivor, Ronald Reagan.

Survivorship has entered the political arena in other ways, with a proliferation of cancer survivor coalitions now jockeying for seats at the public policy table. The survivorship movement began slowly, at the grassroots level, with peer-support groups and programs. Over time, many of these diverse organizations evolved into powerful advocacy groups. Survivors of breast cancer were the first to appreciate and utilize the "squeaky wheel gets the grease" philosophy, and in the process have promoted education and awareness programs, legislation, and advances in screening and treatment procedures. Taking their cue from the highly effective lobbying efforts of AIDS activists, breast cancer survivors banded together in the 1980s to form the National Breast Cancer Coalition. Through their efforts, federal research allocations specifically marked for breast cancer increased

670 percent from 1981 through 1996, from $82 million to $550 million.

Since the 1980s, survivor organizations as diverse as the Candle-lighter's Childhood Cancer Organization, the United Ostomy Association, and the National Prostate Cancer Coalition, to name just a few, have followed suit and successfully rallied Capitol Hill on behalf of their particular cause. Ah, but there's the rub, according to many cancer survivor advocates, myself included. The divergent goals and activities of a fragmented survivorship movement can lead to faction building and a sense of divisiveness. Notes Nancy Davenport-Ennis, executive director of the National Patient Advocate Foundation:

❧ Each specific cancer organization promotes its own separate agenda, and at one time that was a necessary and effective approach. But issues such as job or insurance discrimination, well, those issues affect every cancer patient and survivor, not just those with breast cancer, or lung cancer. To advocate for "body part" legislation ignores the more universal problems faced by every cancer survivor. ❧

There is power in unity, in collective action, in the passion of a purpose. And in the end, the whole will always be greater than the sum of its parts.

Resources for Employment Problems

The agencies and organizations listed below can provide you with additional information about employment discrimination and other work-related issues.

For complaints under Section 503 of the federal Rehabilitation Act, contact:

Office of Federal Contract Compliance Programs
U.S. Department of Labor
200 Constitution Ave., NW, Room C-3325
Washington, D.C. 20210 .
(202) 523-9410

For complaints under Section 504 of the federal Rehabilitation Act, contact:

Department of Health and Human Services
200 Independence Ave., SW
Washington, D.C. 20201
(202) 619-0257

For information about the Americans with Disabilities Act, contact:

U.S. Equal Employment Opportunity Commission
1801 L St., NW
Washington, D.C. 20507
(800) 669-0870 (or 3362)

American Civil Liberties Union (ACLU)
132 West 43rd St.
New York, NY 10036
(212) 944-9800 (or call local listings)
Provides legal assistance for victims of discrimination.

The Cancer Survival Toolbox
(877) TOOLS-4-U (866-5748)
Web site: www.cansearch.org/programs/toolbox.htm
A set of self-learning audiotapes designed to help cancer patients and survivors develop the skills needed to take control of their lives and become stronger self-advocates. Offered free of charge to anyone affected by cancer.

Disability Rights Center
1346 Connecticut Ave., NW
Washington, D.C. 20036
(202) 223-3304

The Job Accommodation Network
(800) 526-7234
A project of the President's Committee on the Employment of People

with Disabilities, this hotline provides information regarding reasonable accommodation.

The National Center for Chronic Disease Prevention
and Health Promotion
Mail Stop K-64
4770 Buford Hwy. NE
Atlanta, GA 30341
(888) 842-6355
Web site: www.cdc.gov/cancer

The National Coalition for Cancer Survivorship (NCCS)
1010 Wayne Ave.
Silver Spring, MD 20910
(301) 565-9670
To order Working It Out: Your Employment Rights as a Cancer
Survivor, *call (301) 650-8868.*

National Patient Advocate Foundation
780 Pilot House Dr., Suite 100-C
Newport News, VA 23606
(757) 873-6668
Web site: www.npaf.org

National Rehabilitation Information Center (NARIC)
U.S. Department of Education
National Institute on Disability Rehabilitation
Research
8455 Colesville Rd., Suite 935
Silver Spring, MD 20910
(800) 34-NARIC (voice/TDD)
*A comprehensive, up-to-date information center and clearinghouse
providing resources and services for disabled people.*

President's Committee on the Employment of
People with Disabilities
1111 20th St., NW
Washington, D.C. 20036
(202) 653-5044
A consortium of individuals and organizations working together to improve the lives and employment opportunities of the disabled.

Rehabilitation Services Administration
Department of Human Services
605 G St., NW
Washington, D.C. 20001
(202) 727-3211
Call for general information on vocational rehabilitation programs in your city, or check your telephone directory under state government listings for your state rehabilitation department.

8
The Double-Edged Sword: Long-Term Effects of Treatment

If I'd known I was going to live this long, I would have taken better care of myself.

— Quentin Crisp

CANCER TREATMENTS keep people alive, but often with undesirable consequences. Most of the unpleasant side effects associated with chemotherapy and radiation can be controlled and eventually will subside once treatment ends. Some effects fade slowly, however, and others may unexpectedly appear months or years later.

Twenty-five years ago, the chief concern facing cancer patients and their doctors was survival; today, quality of life is equally important. Advances in early detection and treatment are controlling malignancies once considered incurable, transforming the public perception of cancer from inexorable terminal illness to serious chronic disease.

Until recently, attention to the long-term and late effects* of cancer treatment wasn't a priority for oncologists, simply because most patients weren't living long enough past diagnosis to be followed. As a result, the focus in cancer care centered on finding more

---

Long-term effects refers to the side effects that persist after treatment ends. *Late effects* are those that occur months or years later.

efficient ways of detecting and treating the disease. Because some of the most significant increases in survival rates in the last thirty years have been in patients with childhood and adolescent cancers, researchers have had the luxury of tracking childhood cancer survivors into adulthood. By documenting their health history, the medical community began to take note of the serious, and in some cases, life-threatening post-treatment complications. With more adults now living longer with the disease, the medical community has expanded the scope of this research to include the adult cancer population. Focused for so long on developing effective therapies to combat cancer, doctors and researchers are at last beginning to take into account the full effect treatment has on the lives they have helped to extend.

Pyrrhic Victories

For some recovered patients, the victory over cancer is in many ways a pyrrhic one. It is not unusual to hear these survivors describe cancer treatment as a double-edged sword, a weapon that damages the patient as it destroys the disease. Cancer treatment can leave them struggling with a variety of disabilities, from chronic pain and disfigurement to organ failure and memory loss. For example, intensive radiation therapy and chemotherapy are highly effective at eradicating Hodgkin's disease in children and adolescents. Because so many of these patients have survived the disease, a great deal is known about post-treatment consequences, such as injury to vital organs and the risk of developing secondary tumors.

Although by comparison my own long-term effects were less severe — a slight limp and chronic lymphedema, or swelling — Lisa, my good friend and cofounder of Cancervive, wasn't so lucky. The aggressive radiation treatment she received for her ovarian cancer caused many serious complications. As you might expect, the issue of long-term effects is of great concern to me, as it is with so many of the survivors I meet.

That is why I thought it important to include this chapter in

Can Survive. I realize that a look at the long-term effects of treatment may come across to some readers as a kind of oncological house of horrors. My intention isn't to scare but rather to alert and inform survivors of some of the latent risks associated with current cancer therapy and to highlight a few treatment-related problems that, with proper follow-up, can be avoided or alleviated.

Unfortunately, some physicians tend to minimize these concerns; they view the lingering and late effects of cancer therapy as the inevitable price of being cured. Newly diagnosed patients, caught up in a climate of stress and urgency, often approach cancer treatment with very little thought to its toxicity. As Deborah Berg, B.S.N., an oncology nurse at the Dana-Farber Cancer Institute, explains:

✎ The oncologist's job is to effectively treat the disease, with the goal of achieving remission. And if subsequent complications arise, then those will be dealt with when they happen. As many of these long- and late-term effects became apparent, the medical community began looking at ways to minimize the damage by modifying treatment. ✎

But not all treatment modifications are safer. The use of new limb-salvage techniques, organ-sparing procedures, gene therapy, and bone marrow transplantations actually increase the complexity of cancer therapy, thereby increasing the potential for serious post-treatment complications.

Surviving cancer is complicated by the fact that today's treatment, although greatly improved over what was available twenty-five years ago, remains an evolving science. It is important for survivors to note that the long-term effects of treatment vary widely and depend on the age of the patient, the type and location of malignancy, the kind of therapy used, and the intensity and duration of that therapy. The more complex and intense a patient's treatment is — for example, a bone marrow or peripheral stem cell transplantation — the greater the chance of late complications. Whereas the effects of surgery are often readily evident, the cumulative effects of chemotherapy and radiation can take years to manifest themselves.

The Long-Term Effects of Chemotherapy

Chemotherapy, as survivors know, involves the use of powerful and, in some cases, toxic chemicals to kill cancer cells. These drugs are often administered in various potent combinations, euphemistically called "chemo cocktails." What makes many anticancer drugs so noxious is that they don't always distinguish between malignant cells and other fast-growing cells that are healthy and normal.

As part of the informed consent procedure when they begin treatment, patients are told that these drugs may have dramatic side effects. And although the immediate consequences are often disturbing, they are measured against the treatment's ability to destroy cancer. Most patients agree that it's a fair trade, so they marshal all their strength and steel themselves for what follows. Once treatment is over, however, they usually expect these side effects to dissipate. Most of them do, but occasionally survivors find they are left with more lasting physical reminders of the battle against cancer. Many of these lingering and late effects can be easily treated, but others pose more serious problems and may even be life-threatening.

Along with thousands of other cancer patients, Alicia, twenty-six, received doxorubicin (Adriamycin) as part of an aggressive chemotherapy regimen for osteosarcoma (bone cancer). Although she is delighted that the treatment seems to have eradicated her cancer, Alicia says she wishes she had been more alert to the possible long-term side effects.

❧ I was sixteen when I was diagnosed and it took all of my strength to get through the chemo. Once I was done, all I wanted was to feel better and get on with living.

I met Rick during my last year at college, and a year later we were married. My health was really never a topic of discussion. I was feeling fine, and I never thought much about cancer anymore.

Rick and I planned on having children, so as soon as we settled down we decided to get started on a family. It didn't take long before I was pregnant. I was fine at first, but by my fifth month, I was beginning to feel extremely weak, with flu-like symptoms. My doctor thought it might have something to do with my hormones kicking up. But it didn't feel like that to me; this seemed different from anything I'd read about in the pregnancy books.

I was worried, but decided that I was probably just having a hard pregnancy. Then one day while I was doing some light exercise, I noticed my heart rate was racing. I started wheezing and I had trouble breathing.

I knew something was definitely wrong. Rick was home so he rushed me to the hospital, where I was pronounced in mild cardiac failure. A physician explained that one of the chemo drugs I'd received, Adriamycin, can be toxic to the heart muscle and the damage can cause problems during periods of extreme stress. I didn't consider exercising to be that stressful, but in my case it was.

I was confined to bed for the duration of my pregnancy and given special heart medication. My labor and delivery were fine, although I was monitored very closely. I gave birth to a healthy baby boy.

My doctor said that none of this would have happened if I had been properly monitored from the start. Since then, I feel as if I've been given a second chance at staying healthy. I now get echocardiograms every year and I make a point to have regular checkups. ॐ

Although Alicia was notified about the possibility of such long-term effects, she admits to never giving it serious consideration. To be sure, some anticancer drugs are more toxic than others and have a greater capacity for inflicting long-term damage on otherwise healthy organs. Both doxorubicin and daunorubicin (Cerubidine), two common antitumor antibiotics, can cause heart damage that in turn may lead to chronic congestive heart failure. The toxicity of these drugs depends on several factors, including the total dose given.

Not every patient treated with these drugs develops later cardiac complications. In fact, patients with strong hearts are at very little risk for cardiotoxicity. Those most at risk include elderly patients (aged seventy or older), patients who have a history of hypertension or coronary heart disease, and those who have received previous irradiation to the chest or were given other drugs that adversely affect the heart. As Alicia learned, congestive heart failure can take years to develop. Once it does, it may come on suddenly. Symptoms include shortness of breath, an inability to tolerate exercise, swelling of the legs and feet, a fast or irregular heartbeat, wheezing, and in some cases chest pain.

To alleviate potential problems, patients who are treated with cardiotoxic drugs are closely monitored throughout treatment. If and when heart damage does occur, many patients respond well to the use of heart medication such as digitalis. Be sure your follow-up exams include an electrocardiogram (EKG) and an echocardiogram, two noninvasive techniques used to assess and monitor heart activity.

There are other drugs that cause later complications: patients who receive bleomycin (Blenoxane) may be at risk for lung fibrosis — the formation of scar tissue in the lungs — which in turn can lead to respiratory problems. The drug cisplatin may cause kidney damage and hearing problems, including tinnitus (ringing in the ears) and hearing loss. The drug vincristine can result in nerve disorders, such as extreme numbness in hands and feet. Many of the chemotherapy drugs classified as alkylating agents (such as cyclophosphamide [Cytoxan] and mechlorethamine) are notable for their ability to damage genetic material.

None of this is intended to suggest that patients who received chemotherapy will necessarily develop post-treatment complications. On the contrary, most bounce back to health and enjoy a life free of serious, treatment-related problems. But it is important to remember that any drug — even aspirin — has the capacity to cause harmful side effects. Good health requires a certain amount of vigilance, and this maxim is doubly true for survivors.

The Long-Term Effects of Radiation

Like chemotherapy, radiation therapy has its own set of acute side effects, most of which are confined to the part of the body being irradiated. Some of the more general short-term complications, such as nausea, skin burns, sores, and hair loss, subside shortly after treatment ends. As with chemotherapy, however, sometimes these complications are permanent, whereas others don't manifest themselves until much later.

When thirty-two-year-old Jose-Luis first noticed symptoms of a glioblastoma (brain tumor) seven years ago, he was working as a certified public accountant for a large accounting firm. He underwent surgery to remove the tumor as well as six weeks of cranial radiation and chemotherapy. But several months into recovery, Jose-Luis realized that he was having treatment-related difficulties. He explains what happened:

&⁷ I encountered a problem one day when I sat down to write a few checks. Right away, I saw that I was having trouble doing simple calculations. I thought that maybe I was somehow off that day, and that I probably needed to take it easy. But a couple of months later, I was still having difficulties.

To someone trained as an accountant, the loss of such basic skills is upsetting, to put it mildly. My doctor suggested I see a psychologist, who then put me through a battery of tests. I learned a lot from those evaluation tests on how radiation had affected my thinking process. One test revealed that I had difficulty putting things in sequence, another pointed to memory problems. I called my neurologist and asked him what was going on. He informed me that my problems were probably caused by the radiation. He said I'd received the maximum dose and that it may have caused permanent damage.

Since then, as a result of the radiation, I've done a few really strange things. I remember going to a dinner party with some friends not too long ago. There was a bottle of champagne on the dinner table and next to it an empty champagne bucket. I stared at these two objects for a while, then picked up the bottle, opened it, and proceeded to empty it into the bucket. Everyone at the party watched in stunned silence. It took me a few minutes to realize what I had done, and then I was tremendously embarrassed. At the time it just seemed to make perfect sense. I now know that the radiation treatment had scrambled my thinking process. Fortunately, these little incidents don't happen too often. ❧

Thanks to impressive advances in radiation therapy (including radium implants, gamma knife, etc.) this type of treatment is now an effective weapon against certain types of formerly fatal brain tumors. But to achieve remission, high doses of radiation to the head are necessary. What is it then about this kind of treatment that causes such changes in the thinking process? Dr. Jordan Wilbur, chief of pediatric oncology at Children's Cancer Research Institute at the Pacific Presbyterian Medical Center in San Francisco, explains: "In many ways the brain is like a computer. Each thought process involves millions of neural connections. As a result of cranial radiation, some of the neural connections that deal with understanding certain concepts can 'burn out'; they simply don't connect anymore. In very young patients, those under age five or six, this is invariably the case. With older patients, it depends on how much radiation is involved."

As with chemotherapy, radiation batters normal body tissue while it goes about its mission of destroying cancer cells. Consequently, patients who receive irradiation to the head or the central nervous system frequently experience a minor decrease in I.Q. level and attention span and are at risk for other problems involving perception and motor skills. As Dr. Wilbur notes, young children are particularly vulnerable to later radiation-caused learning disabilities. Fortunately, many of these problems are remediable and can be corrected with early intervention.

The long-term effects of any radiation treatment depend on location and dosage. Irradiation of the chest, for example, can lead to permanent scarring of the lungs. Children who receive high-dose radiation to the head and skeletal system may later develop problems with physical development. When the head is irradiated, the part of the brain that produces growth hormone, the pituitary gland, can be affected, resulting in a diminished growth rate. Radiotherapy to the spine, abdomen, or pelvis may also result in restricted growth. During follow-up, physicians monitor such children and refer them to an endocrinologist if problems develop.

Intense radiotherapy can cause a multitude of other late complications, more than I can possibly list here. Again, it is your responsibility to learn about the potential problems that may result from your type of treatment and to discuss any late effect concerns with your oncologist.

Lymphedema

In many patients, radiation or surgery can damage or destroy healthy lymph nodes and channels, resulting in chronic swelling. This condition is called lymphedema and is the result of the lymphatic system's inability to rid itself of accumulated lymph fluid. Most commonly lymphedema develops in an arm or a leg, although, depending on where radiation or surgery occurred, other parts of the body can be affected.

The swelling associated with lymphedema occurs when an abnormal amount of this protein-rich lymph fluid collects and stagnates in the affected area. Normally functioning lymph nodes and the channels that connect them act as a filtering system against bacteria and other impurities in the body. Left untreated, lymphedema may disrupt the job of this filtering system, leaving the affected limb susceptible to infection (lymphangitis) and other sometimes irreversible complications. Lymphedema may occur at any time, from a few days to a few years after surgery or treatment. For some, the condition is mild and painless, seemingly no more than a cosmetic nuisance. For others, it can develop into a major source of discomfort, disability, and shame.

I first noticed the telltale signs of lymphedema three years after my treatment for rhabdomyosarcoma when my ankle and later my entire right leg began to swell. My doctor informed me that high-dose radiation to my right thigh had resulted in fibrosis, causing these adhesions of connective tissue to block lymphatic channels. Although the condition seemed innocuous at first, I've occasionally experienced recurring infections (cellulitis) in my right leg as a result of a minor cut or abrasion. Following years of trial and error, I've found that the most effective treatment for lymphedema is lymph massage, together with the use of a compression stocking.

For Iris, a forty-eight-year-old airline executive, lymphedema came on quite unexpectedly. Four years ago, she was found to have a small malignant lump in her right breast. She chose to have a lumpectomy, followed by lymph node dissection (the removal of lymph nodes surrounding the tumor). All nodes tested negative, but her oncologist suggested a course of radiation as a protective measure.

✎ Other than the fatigue, I experienced no real problems with the radiation sessions. But I was becoming increasingly concerned about my arm. It continued to feel heavy and wooden. Then one night I started getting dressed for a party. It was the first time since my cancer treatment that I'd worn a long-sleeved dress. I knew something was wrong when I tried to get my right arm through the sleeve and it wouldn't fit. My first thought was, Oh my God. It's the cancer. It's back!

My doctor referred me to a physical therapist, who in turn measured me for a compression sleeve. I was also advised not to injure the arm in any way, that even an insect bite to the area could cause serious infection.

I hated the idea of having a chronically swollen arm. Since I was under the impression that nothing could be done, I ignored the swelling for a long time.

But all that changed when my arm did indeed become seriously infected. I had to be hospitalized, and to make a long story short, it scared me into taking action. Not long after that, I attended a local lymphedema support group. The physical therapist there emphasized that if my lymphedema was not managed, the stagnant fluid would eventually cause the tissue in my arm to harden and would limit my mobility.

I left the meeting relieved yet still angry that treatment for cancer had left me with such a disfiguring and potentially dangerous side effect. I'm still wondering why I wasn't given more information early on about how to manage it. ❧

If, like Iris, you have undergone cancer treatment that involved radiation or node dissection, you may be at risk for lymphedema. Precautionary steps include:

- *Protect the limb from any cuts or burns.* Protection requires special attention on your part, such as avoiding sunburn, using an electric razor instead of a blade for shaving, and wearing gloves during gardening or while doing the dishes. Insect or animal bites to the affected limb require prompt medical attention. Even something as innocuous as cutting your cuticles can result in infection.

- *Keep abrasions clean.* If the skin is cut or broken in any way, wash the area immediately with soap and water, apply antibacterial medication, and cover with a bandage.

- *Have doctors or nurses use only your unaffected arm for injections, IV's, and blood pressure readings.* Again, any kind of trauma to the affected area can create a problem. It's a good idea to carry with you a special medical ID tag identifying your impaired limb (see p. 181).

- *Watch out for pressure and fluid retention.* Keep clothing and jewelry loose to avoid pressure. Also, try to reduce or maintain your weight to lessen pressure on the lymph system.

- *Elevate the limb.* Rest the affected limb in an elevated position whenever possible to relieve swelling.

- *Exercise with moderation.* As important as it is to be careful of your impaired arm or leg, that doesn't mean you should baby it. Keep muscle tone up through regular exercise (including postmastectomy exercises), but do avoid overexerting or stressing the limb. Recommended exercise programs include light aerobics, swimming, walking, and yoga. To be on the safe side, consult with your doctor or a physical therapist before beginning any new exercise program.

- *Wear a compression garment.* To keep swelling in check, wear a compression garment over the affected limb during the day. Be sure to have the fit checked periodically (every four to six months is advisable). Be especially attentive about wearing the garment and any additionally recommended wrapped bandages during long airplane flights.

- *Watch for warning signals.* Contact your physician immediately if the affected area turns red or becomes blistered, tender, or painful.

- *Wear a medical tag.* In the event of an accident or emergency, a LYMPHEDEMA ALERT bracelet will tip off medical personnel to your condition and could quite possibly save your affected limb from the kind of poking and prodding that can trigger lymphedema, exacerbate an existing case, or lead to an infection. The bracelet clearly states "LYMPHEDEMA ALERT: No Blood Pressure — No Needles in [the affected area]." The bracelet can be ordered through the National Lymphedema Network (see p. 184).

As Iris discovered, there is no cure for lymphedema, but treatments to control its symptoms do exist. Camilla B. Fiore, R.N., is an oncology nurse who has extensively studied lymphedema and ways of controlling it. She notes: "The most significant barrier to people seeking effective treatment is the negative effect lymphedema has on self-esteem. Teenagers in particular have a tough time dealing with it. I recently saw a young man who had deferred treatment for leg lymphedema until it had moved into his groin. You can do so much to control the condition if you catch it early. Why wait until it's a real problem?"

Fiore recommends Complex Decongestive Physiotherapy (CDP) as the most effective therapy for lymphedema at present. CDP is a four-step treatment process that includes manual lymphatic drainage, a gentle manual stimulation of the skin to break up, or decongest, lymph fluid in underlying soft tissue, followed by the use of a custom bandage or compression garment to reduce fibrosis and aid in lymph fluid circulation.

Vasopneumatic pressure pumps are considered by some to be an effective tool for managing mild edema-like swelling, but Fiore does not recommend their use for lymphedema. "I think pumps work up to a point, but are much less efficient in managing lymphedema than manual lymphatic drainage." She also warns against the use of benzopyrones, a class of drugs available in Europe to treat lymphedema, as their efficacy and safety remain in question.

Fiore emphasizes that the technique of manual lymphatic drainage has yet to be standardized in this country, so those seeking this treatment should decline services from anyone other than a physical therapist certified in MLD training. And beware of a therapist who quotes you the cost of a session over the phone; lymphedema is a medical condition that requires professional evaluation and followup. An MLD therapist should have a minimum of 135 hours of certified training by a specialist from one of the following schools.

Dr. Vodder School (Victoria, British Columbia, Canada)
Web site: www.voderschool.com

The Foldi Clinic (Germany)
Web site: www.foeldiklink.de

Academy of Lymphatic Studies (Sebastian, Florida)
Lerner Lymphedema Services
Web site: www.gate.net/~vda/academy.html

The cost of Manual Lymphatic Drainage currently runs from $250 to $350 per session; the number of sessions required will depend on the severity of your condition. Treatment for lymphedema is not always covered by insurance, although a 1998 law now mandates that insurance companies covering for breast reconstructive surgery after mastectomy must also cover lymphedema treatment.

Compression garments are not always covered by insurance. Contact your insurance company to find out what your plan allows. These are retailers for support sleeves and stockings.

Beiersdorf, Inc. Bandages and Padding
BDF Plaza
Norwalk, CT 06856
(800) 876-3664 (x805)

Beiersdorf-Jobst, Inc.
5825 Carnegie Blvd.
Charlotte, NC 28209
(704) 554-9933 or (704) 551-7189
For pumps and ready-made and custom-fit compression garments. Ask about Elvarex stockings.

Circaid Medical Products
9323 Chesapeake Dr.
Suite B-2
San Diego, CA 92123
(800) CIRCAID or (619) 576-3550
e-mail: infor@circaid.com
Web site: www.circaid.com

Juzo Compression Products
(a.k.a. Julius Zorn, Inc.)
P.O. Box 1088
80 Chart Rd.
Cuyahoga Falls, OH 44223
(800) 222-4999

e-mail: juzousa@aol.com
Web site: www.juzo.com

Legacy Directional Flow Compression System
1800 NW Market St.
Suite 219
Seattle, WA 98107
(206) 782-8554

Medi Stockings and Sleeves
76 West Seegers Rd.
Arlington Heights, IL 60005
(800) 633-6334

Peninsula Medical
P.O. Box 7317
Standford, CA 94309
(800) 29-EDEMA
e-mail: edemarx@aol.com
Supplier of the Reid sleeve.

Sigvaris
P.O. Box 570
32 Park Drive East
Branford, CT 06405
(800) 322-7744

For further information on the treatment of lymphedema, contact the National Lymphedema Network, a nonprofit resource center: 2211 Post St., Suite 404, San Francisco, CA 94115; (800) 541-3259. Web site: www.lymphnet.org.

Chronic Fatigue

Fatigue is one of the hallmarks of cancer therapy, and the most common. Patients expect radiation or chemotherapy to play havoc with their stamina. Fighting off a life-threatening disease is, after all, exhausting work. But once treatment ends, patients look forward to regaining all their hard-spent energy. Instead, months or even years later, they may find that they're still feeling run down, mustering all their strength just to get through the day. Cancer treatment–related fatigue can be such a problem for some survivors — particularly those who have undergone bone marrow transplantation — that they find it hard to function at a normal level.

Jane Hawgood, a clinical social worker at the University of California–San Francisco Medical Center and a long-term survivor of breast cancer, notes that the medical community used to pass fatigue off as a sign of depression, but they now realize that in many cases there are organic reasons for it.

Hawgood adds that low blood count, emotional stress, and nutritional deficiencies are all considered possible culprits for causing fatigue. Some believe it is brought about by the additional energy the body must expend on rebuilding injured cells. Others suspect that bone marrow suppression is responsible. After treatment, bone marrow recovery may be slow or incomplete, which in turn inhibits the production of infection-fighting white blood cells, oxygen-carrying red blood cells, and blood-clotting platelets. If the white blood cell count drops below normal, the body has to use more energy to fight infection and repair damaged cells; if the red blood cell count is too low, anemia can result.

Since the cancer experience is so emotionally draining and disruptive to a person's lifestyle, many physicians believe that a patient's lack of pep is caused by depression. To be sure, fatigue and listlessness are often the physical counterparts of grief or depression. If you think your lack of energy could have psychological roots, you may want to get in touch with a support group or therapist. For some people, emotion-based fatigue is a temporary state; they learn to recognize why they are feeling low and find ways to pull themselves through the down times. For others, depression is a more deep-seated problem and therefore requires more serious attention.

"Many survivors find that coming to terms with fatigue means changing their lifestyle to fit their diminished energy level," explains Hawgood. "It may require accepting a new 'normal' level of activity." She adds that survivors who are struggling with chronic fatigue might want to consider the following suggestions:

- *Listen to your body; understand your fatigue.* Try to understand when you are most likely to be affected by fatigue, then look for ways of managing it. Find time to take short naps or breaks. (But don't take it too easy; excessive bed rest weakens the body.) If naps don't suit you, experiment with other kinds of relaxation. Some survivors report that it helps to spend quiet time alone, meditating, reading, or writing in a journal.

- *Try to organize your day so that you conserve as much energy as possible.* Determine what the most productive time of the day is for you and gauge yourself accordingly.

- *Don't try to do the impossible.* Some survivors attempt to maintain their old schedules and routines, then feel frustrated because they run out of steam before they've accomplished what they set out to do. Prioritize your day and conserve your energy for essential tasks. Accept that your lack of energy is treatment-related and don't try to fight it. But don't let it defeat you either.

- *Maintain a healthy diet and exercise program.* If you aren't eating a well-balanced, nutritional diet, you're bound to feel run down sooner or later. Food is fuel. Make sure that the foods you eat provide you with the nourishment you need to maintain strength and energy. And don't overlook the importance of regular exercise as an antidote to low energy and an outlet for emotions. Exercise is an excellent way to build up strength and stamina after treatment.

- *Have a physical examination.* To rule out any medical causes, schedule an appointment with your doctor for a complete physical. Anemia, hypothyroidism, or an infection could be contributing to your fatigue, and should be promptly treated.

To learn more about cancer treatment–related fatigue, contact the Oncology Nursing Society's Web site at www.cancerfatigue.org.

The Risk of Secondary Tumors

Although the fear of recurrence lurks in the back of most survivors' minds, few give much thought to the chance of new or secondary tumors. Current research indicates that approximately five percent of survivors may develop a secondary cancer. Factors influencing the chances include genetic tendencies (i.e., a family disposition for a certain form of cancer), lifestyle habits (smoking, excessive alcohol consumption), radiation treatment, or the use of certain chemotherapy agents, such as Cytoxan, Ifosfamide, Melphalan, or Etoposide. The possibility of secondary tumors should be of special concern to survivors of childhood cancer, who are surviving longer and are therefore at greater risk for developing late complications of their treatments. Because cancer patients in general are living longer, those survivors who were treated with high-dose chemotherapy and radiation should be aware of the need to monitor for treatment-related secondary cancers. Non-Hodgkin's lymphoma survivors, for instance, show an increased risk for developing myelodysplastic syndrome — an abnormality of the bone marrow considered a form of preleukemia — five or ten years out from treatment.

I recently met a thirty-six-year-old survivor who knows all about those risks. Carla is a free-lance artist who was diagnosed at age one with Wilms' tumor, a form of kidney cancer that primarily affects children. In the mid-'50s, treatment for Wilms' included surgery (in Carla's case, to remove her left kidney), followed by intensive radiation and chemotherapy. The treatment worked and her cancer was eradicated. But as Carla explains, she's been struggling with the consequences of that cure ever since.

&? My parents didn't tell me I had cancer until I was twelve. Even then, I never really got the details. Families deal with cancer in different ways. My family chose to deal with it by not dealing with it. By the time I was a teenager, I had become very angry and resentful that my family had handled my illness the way they did. For example, the radiation had affected growth on the left side of my torso. It also left me with a curved spine. A lot of things that could have been done in the way of reconstructive surgery were just never addressed.

I was thirty years old when, during a follow-up visit, I told my doctor about a hard lump I'd found in my right breast. I wasn't really worried about it though. I'd had many benign lumps removed over the years — from my breasts, my bladder, my back, you name it. So I thought this was probably just another noncancerous growth. Since I hadn't been warned about the risk of future secondary malignancies, I never considered cancer to be a possibility. I actually believed that since I'd already had the disease, I was safe.

When the doctor told me my breast lump was malignant, I refused to believe her. I went for a second opinion, and then a third. But there was no getting around it; I had cancer again. All the doctors said that the tumor "looked good" — I love that expression — and that other than a mastectomy, I wouldn't need any further treatment. Now that I think of it, I was still in denial right up to the time of the operation.

While I was recovering, my doctor explained how my early treatment for Wilms' may have precipitated this tumor and that I could very well be at risk for further breast cancer. She gave me more information about late effects than I had ever received in my life. My doctor gave me the choice of whether to continue with intensive follow-ups and early mammograms or have the other breast removed as a precautionary measure. She wasn't pushy, but she strongly urged me to consider a second mastectomy.

My first reaction was "Forget it! I'd rather die than go through that." It was just too much too soon. I told my doctor I needed to think about it. And I did, for a year. I spent a lot of that year feeling sorry for myself. During this time I also had to deal with early menopause, another late effect. I was carrying around a lot of anger and resentment, and I didn't want to deal with the very real possibility of finding another malignant lump in my breast. It's a stupid attitude, I know. But that's how I felt.

It took me a long time to get beyond all that. I thought long and hard about it and finally realized that I was looking at a possible life-or-death decision. I went ahead with the operation and later had breast reconstruction surgery.

The surgeon told me the tissue in that breast was precancerous, so I guess I made the right decision. But it wasn't easy. It was a major process for me to go from bitterness and complete denial to active decision making.

My attitude has totally changed since that second mastectomy. I'm much more assertive now about my health. ❧

The great irony of cancer treatment is that the methods used to eradicate cancer can also lay the ground for future malignancies. Radiation, like certain chemotherapy drugs belonging to the alkylating group, can potentially cause a variety of secondary cancers, including leukemia, bone sarcomas, and thyroid cancer. Studies show that while the majority of survivors will remain free of their initial disease, their chances of contracting another cancer are about three times higher than that of the rest of the population.

This isn't to imply that cancer therapy is inadvisable. On the contrary, the efficacy of current forms of treatment cannot be underestimated. Without them there would undoubtedly be fewer treatment complications and far fewer survivors. Half a million people are successfully treated for cancer each year, and of that number, only a small percentage is at risk for treatment-induced malignancies.

Then again, not all relapses and secondary cancers are the result of treatment. Genetic tendencies and lifestyle habits, such as smoking and excessive sun exposure, also play a role in whether a survivor will develop a secondary cancer. The study of long-term effects of treatment is so new that doctors still have difficulty identifying symptoms that are treatment-related and those that would have occurred regardless of therapy.

Survivors need to remember that most secondary tumors can be successfully controlled if caught early. Annual checkups at a long-term follow-up clinic, preferably by a physician familiar with your cancer history, should be an important part of your life.

As Dr. Maurie Markman, a medical oncologist at the Cleveland Clinic Cancer Center, observes: "It is critical for survivors to know about the risks and to be vigilant, and it would be great if we could completely avoid the side effects. But don't forget that the goal of cancer treatment is to keep people alive."

When Anger Becomes a Long-Term Effect

The emotional storm created by cancer doesn't necessarily end with treatment. Rather, as a survivor, you are faced with new concerns, new challenges, and many more questions. What, if any, long-term effects will you encounter? If surgery has altered your appearance or self-image, how will you learn to accept this new you? How can you best handle the anger and frustration over all the changes cancer has created in your life? The process of sorting through these issues can be a big job, one that many survivors approach with a great deal of bitterness. As Carla says: "Most of us thought that the worst was over once treatment ended. For many of us it isn't, and yet we're supposed to grin and bear it."

A presumption long held by both the medical community and the population at large was that remission was reward enough for the cancer patient. Gratitude, not grief or anger, was considered the proper response. And while you undoubtedly are grateful, there may be other, unanticipated emotions. You may feel embarrassed or guilty about the anger you are feeling. You might even think you aren't entitled to these emotions. I know I felt that way after I developed lymphedema. Once I was free of cancer, everyone expected me to be beyond any emotional pain or resentment over the side effects I suffered. But that is so much easier said than done.

Jose-Luis, the former accountant introduced earlier in this chapter, also continues to wrestle with the emotional and physical aftermath of cancer therapy for his brain tumor.

๛ The most difficult part of my recovery was adjusting to the effects of treatment and the anger it has generated. Since my cancer I've become totally dependent on my family for everything. I am unable to return to my former line of work. My depth perception and motor skills have been affected to the point where I can no longer drive a car. My life is so different now, and some days that's very hard for me to accept.

I'm angry that I never got the full picture from my doctors on how treatment might affect me. I'm sure that I would have still gone through with it and taken my chances, but at least I would have felt that it was a shared decision. When you haven't been warned, and then all of a sudden these things come out of left field and turn your life upside down, it's terribly discouraging. Once you stop feeling sorry for yourself, you get depressed and angry. And sometimes you stay that way.

Therapy has helped me to learn how to find an outlet for my anger. I'm also taking special education classes every day for some of the problems treatment caused, and that's helped me refocus my thoughts. I enjoy swimming, so when I'm feeling upset, I'll go for a long swim and that relieves some of the stress. Other times, I'll simply close the door to my room and scream and yell for a few minutes. ๛

Some illnesses are fairly easy to put behind us, but cancer isn't one of them. Once you've been diagnosed, cancer becomes a piece of your identity, a part of your life. If the disease or its treatment has created physical disabilities or altered your body image, the psychological residue can include a profound sense of unfairness and anger.

And as Carla and Jose-Luis discovered, those emotions can be very hard to assuage.

Finding Ways to Take Charge of Anger

Barbara J. Carter, a mental health registered nurse and research scientist who has studied the issues of cancer survivorship extensively, states that anger is healthy, provided you use it productively: "Anger acts like a signpost; it signifies that something important has happened to us, and it should be heeded. The best way to deal with anger is to find a constructive outlet for it. Get it to work for you, not against you."

I have found, as have many survivors, that the best way to come to grips with anger — or any strong emotion for that matter — is to face it head-on. This may be frightening to you, even unacceptable. Carter notes that many of us learn from an early age to keep a lid on our emotions, especially volatile ones like anger. Others view the expression of anger as a sign of weakness, or as a violation of good manners. However, if you cannot find a way to let off steam, your anger may eventually lead to explosive outbursts that have the potential to damage relationships. Be kind to yourself and others. Give yourself permission to ask for help in handling your anger.

For many people, anger most often takes the form of blame or self-reproach. Some of the angriest survivors are those who, like Carla and Jose-Luis, were never told that they might have problems as a result of treatment.

Jose-Luis, for instance, says that because no one informed him that his radiation therapy might lead to short-term memory loss, his recovery was doubly frustrating.

ॐ It took me months to figure out that my memory problems were due to treatment. It is an incredibly odd sensation, feeling like you've lost some of your brain power. The resulting anger caused me to be hard on myself. Then I found out through a support group that many other survivors who have received radiation to the head suffered from similar problems. We shared experiences, swapped stories, and even laughed about it. As a consequence, I don't beat myself up so much anymore. ॐ

Dr. Patricia Ganz, a medical oncologist and professor at the University of California–Los Angeles, observes:

ॐ Studies show that many survivors of childhood malignancies were never even told they were treated for cancer. They had no way of knowing later on why they were having learning difficulties or problems with physical growth. Their anger is understandable. It may help allay a lot of anxiety for these survivors to know that there are legitimate medical reasons for their problems.

Then again, some survivors say, "I was never told about these things," when in fact they *are* told what to expect before treatment begins, but they just don't hear it. They are engulfed in fear and so focused on getting through treatment that they block it out. Then when these problems surface later on, there is an initial sense of shock, followed by strong feelings of anger and resentment. ॐ

Even those patients who have the presence of mind to absorb and accept the potential risks involved may react bitterly when complications occur. They find themselves overwhelmed with strong feelings of anger and resentment toward their physicians, toward life, even toward their own bodies for betraying them. Says Grace Christ, professor at Columbia University's School of Social Work, "I think some of the frustration survivors feel is due in part to the difficulty they have getting doctors to pay attention to their post-treatment concerns. Some oncologists find it hard to address the topic of late effects. Their daily preoccupation revolves around trying to save lives."

Some recovered patients find the only way they can resolve their emotional turmoil is by communicating how they feel to their physicians. Find time when you can both sit down and calmly discuss the repercussions of your treatment. Such an exchange may put to rest some of your resentment and anger and help speed your emotional recovery.

Years ago, Lisa and I decided to pay a visit to the radiation therapist who had treated us at Stanford University Medical Center. We went looking for answers to the many questions we had about the late effects of radiotherapy. We also wanted to vent our frustration over how treatment complications had affected our lives. As you might imagine, it was a very emotional meeting and, to our surprise, very cathartic.

Of course, if you choose to have this kind of discussion with your doctor, bear in mind that it may not go the way you planned. Some doctors simply aren't comfortable discussing patients' emotional problems. Also, be aware that you and your doctor are likely to have different perceptions of your cancer experience, so don't expect to see eye to eye on everything. Try to gauge how open your physician is to what you have to say. If your doctor is not responsive to your concerns, don't hesitate to find one who is.

Whatever actions you choose to pursue, try to funnel your anger into a productive way of taking care of your needs. That is what Carla did.

&8 I don't know if I'll ever stop feeling bitter over what happened to me, but at least I've found a way to handle it. I've been going to support group meetings for the past year, and that kind of networking has been a big help. When I'm with the group I can express all that pain and frustration with people who've been there. I've learned how to use visualization techniques, positive thinking, all that stuff. I've also pulled my head out of the sand. Now I make sure that I'm as informed and as knowledgeable as possible whenever I'm faced with an important decision. I've really taken it upon myself to be my own advocate, and that's helped me to be stronger and more confident about myself. &8

The Importance of Follow-Up

No one is immune to illness; everyone is at some risk of getting cancer. But as a survivor, you live with heightened risks. That is why comprehensive follow-up exams are so important. But Dr. Frank Meyskens, Jr., director of the Chow Cancer Center at the University of California–Irvine, has observed that more than a few survivors prefer to ignore follow-ups: "Some recovered patients don't want to be reminded of their disease and so they avoid regular checkups. Those are the people who will be more at risk for later problems. Concerned survivors, on the other hand, are going to be more active in their health care and will have a much better chance of catching problems early on."

If returning to "the scene of the crime" gives you the creeps, talk it over with a member of your health care team or with another survivor. It might help if you remind yourself that medical checkups are preventive medicine, indeed, the best possible insurance for your newfound health. They also provide you with an opportunity to touch base with your physician, ask questions, and catch up on any late-breaking news regarding your type of cancer. Remember that even though checkup exams are hard on your nerves, they can also be an important source of reassurance, with negative test results providing you with a clean bill of health.

But that's not all. Not only are your checkups valuable for safeguarding your health, but they also provide the medical community with documentation of possible long-term effects. That is why it is important to continue your follow-up visits at the hospital or institution that originally treated you. Your feedback during checkups will facilitate further modification of treatment for future patients.

The responsibility for follow-up care doesn't lie solely with survivors; the medical community must also take a more active role in attending to the long-term needs of recovered cancer patients. However, the current emphasis on managed care, with its preoccupation with cost containment, discourages patient referrals to specialists for adequate follow-up care. Susan Leigh, a registered nurse who serves as a board member with the National Coalition for Cancer Survivorship, believes the medical community has been slow to address the long-term health concerns of survivors: "Not enough hospitals offer any real rehabilitation programs for cancer patients. Cardiac patients, who have a much higher chance of dying from their disease than do cancer patients, have all kinds of comprehensive rehabilitation programs in place. We're losing people through the current system because many survivors just aren't coming back for their yearly checkups. Survivors should have physical exams that are tailored to their specific needs. Instead, most survivors are having to formulate their own health maintenance programs."

Years, even decades, after recovery, you should still consider yourself a key member of your treatment team. Also, if you haven't already done so, find ways of making your life healthier, whether that means altering your diet or looking into stress-reduction techniques. Even the smallest changes can have far-reaching effects. It might help if you think of your body as a finely tuned machine. Doctors can perform maintenance checks and overhauls, but it's your job to look after the daily upkeep.

Resources for Survivor Wellness

Many hospitals and medical centers around the country have established late-effects clinics within their oncology departments. That these centers exist is an auspicious indication that the medical community is beginning to accommodate the need for long-term follow-up of cancer survivors. Because most survivorship research has focused on the pediatric cancer population, however, these clinics are primarily geared toward young survivors. Recovered patients of any age may nevertheless consult with the late-effects specialists who are affiliated with these clinics.

Childhood Cancer Survivors

Survivors of childhood cancer should check with the cancer center where they were treated for information on long-term follow-up clinics or programs in your area. The following are two such long-standing programs.

Children's Hospital of Los Angeles
4650 Sunset Blvd.
Los Angeles, CA 90027
(213) 660-2450
The hospital offers a Long-Term Information, Follow-up, and Evaluation Program (LIFE), which provides education and psychosocial support to adult survivors of childhood cancer.

Dream Street Camp
The nonprofit Dream Street Foundation sponsors a summer camp each year at Canyon Ranch in Tucson, Arizona, for teens and young adults who have experienced a life-threatening illness.
1-800-55-DREAM

Post-Treatment Resource Program
Memorial Sloan-Kettering Cancer Center
410 East 62nd St.
New York, NY 10021
(212) 639-3292
Web site: www.cure.acor.org
The Association of Cancer Online Resources, Inc. (ACOR) offers scores of Internet support groups, such as PED-ONC, a GVHD support group for post-BMT patients, and BMT-TALK.

Adult Survivors

For the most up-to-date research information into the physical and psychosocial issues facing cancer survivors, contact:

> The National Cancer Institute
> Office of Cancer Survivorship
> 6130 Executive Blvd.
> Bethesda, MD 20890
> (301) 496-4000

In addition to long-term effects clinics, former cancer patients may want to look into survivor-oriented wellness programs now offered by health spas, cruise lines, and resorts around the country.

Living with Compromise

Recovery from cancer often involves adjusting to changes in one's physical appearance and abilities. You may have endured a visible loss, an amputation, extensive scarring, loss of mobility. Or your loss may be less obvious, affecting your ability to be an athlete or a math whiz. Part of you has been altered, and as a result you may feel diminished, no longer the same person. Moving out of the treatment phase and on to the rest of your life entails assimilating this "new you," tailoring your expectations to who you are now.

More than two decades after my own cancer treatment, I still find it difficult to accept that I limp. Walking past a store window, I have trouble identifying with the reflection I see. The image doesn't jibe with the "me" still preserved in my mind's eye, the me that knows what it feels like to run, to ski, to be, quite literally, fast on my feet. In time I learned to integrate this change into a new sense of self. I found ways to come to terms with what I had lost and acknowledge that the loss was beyond my control, and I managed to get on with the job of living.

Cancer researcher Barbara Carter notes, "Because of permanent physical alterations, some survivors will continue to live out their cancer experience for the rest of their lives. Humpty Dumpty can never be the same again."

The "Humpty Dumpty syndrome" is in fact an apt description of the post-treatment cancer patient. Dr. Fitzhugh Mullan, co-founder of the National Coalition for Cancer Survivorship and himself a survivor, uses this phrase to describe how a recovering patient strives to regain a sense of normality after cancer, to piece life back together again. Eventually the survivor learns to accept that the pieces may not fit the way they did before.

How do you come to terms with this newly reconstructed view of yourself? Many survivors find that physical or occupational therapy gives them the assistance they need to readapt comfortably. Sometimes physical rehabilitation, such as breast reconstruction, can be a positive step toward accepting a new body image. Of course, restorative rehabilitation is no magic act. It isn't going to improve every aspect of your life automatically. But it may very well improve your self-image, and that can make a big difference in how you approach life. Barbara Carter adds, "When your body undergoes a dramatic change, you need to completely revamp your self-image, and that isn't easy. First you need to work through the grieving process and accept the loss of your former self. Once you've allowed that to happen, you can begin to reconstitute a new view of yourself through the cancer experience. A part of that process involves the reactions and support of other people, especially family and friends. By coming to terms with the feelings of friends and loved ones and infusing them with your own, you can slowly start to reassemble a new self-image."

Roaring down the road of recovery, years after their cancer experience, most survivors still find themselves glancing in the rearview mirror, checking out where they've been and who they've become. This process of integrating a new body image — that is, coming to terms with the physical aspects of the cancer experience — can take a long time, sometimes a lifetime. If that's happening to you, consider it normal; acceptance comes in small increments. Survivor Jane Hawgood found this to be true for herself.

&b You may need lots of time to mourn the physical loss, whether it's your prostate, your breast, your hair, or your former stamina. You have to experience the shock and the grief, the sadness and the anger, before you can get to the point where you can then say, "Okay. This is how it is. Now let's get on with life." With some losses, like mastectomies, it can take even longer to get to that point. I know that a lot of women say, as I did, "Hey, I'm okay. It really doesn't bother me." But it does. We put on a brave face because we feel a lot of pressure to be normal again. It can be especially hard to come to terms with your loss if the people around you are denying it. It's up to you to push beyond that denial, ask for their support, and find ways of reaffirming your own positive perceptions of who you are. &b

Three years after the discovery of her lymphedema, Iris has learned how to adjust to what she calls her "oversized arm."

&b It used to be painful for me to even look at my right arm. Sometimes it would get so swollen it looked deformed. I would try to hide it under loose clothing or just pretend that it didn't exist. Deep down, I knew I was rejecting this part of my body because it was cosmetically unappealing. A serious infection woke me up to the fact that by ignoring my lymphedema I was jeopardizing my life. In the end, I realized that by taking responsibility for my lymphedema I also took ownership of it. &b

Carla says that by accepting the physical changes brought about by cancer, she has become a much stronger person.

&b All of the coping I've done has really steeled me, made me a lot tougher. I'm more in control of my life now than I have ever been. I'll admit, sometimes depression will come creeping up on me. I'll start feeling sorry for myself and then get angry. At the end of the day, it just wears me down. That's when I'll hightail it to a support group meeting. If that's not possible, I'll call up Mimi, a friend I met through the group. Mimi has gone through three bouts of cancer since she was a child, and like me, she's had a double mastectomy. Unlike me, she's been able to fully separate her sense of self-worth from the physical damage and uses humor and a self-deprecating wit to fend off bitterness. Through her, I've begun to realize how important it is to consider each new day as a gift and to recognize the therapeutic value of laughter. &8

9

The Cycle of Life: Sexuality and Fertility After Cancer

AT THE CORE of the cancer survivor's experience is the concept of loss: loss of innocence and security, loss of physical integrity, loss of hopes and dreams. However, of all the necessary losses caused by cancer treatment, perhaps none is as poignant as the loss of fertility. Surgery, chemotherapy, radiation, and hormone therapy can play havoc with a cancer patient's reproductive system. Fortunately, for many this effect is usually temporary. For some, though, the potential for future life is lost in the battle to sustain one's own life.

Cancer complicates issues of sexuality as well. Physical and psychological changes brought about by treatment — alterations ranging from diminished stamina or libido to the loss of a body part and damaged self-image — can give rise to a host of sexual problems. Single survivors of any age, including those divorced or widowed, often emerge from treatment with high anxiety and deep doubts about their sexual appeal and their ability to sustain lasting relationships. Even those in long-term stable relationships may encounter unanticipated problems related to sexual desire, sexual functioning, and intimacy. Most often, these problems are experienced by those with breast, colorectal, genitourinary, or gynecological cancers, although any form of the disease has the potential of interfering with sexual health and function.

According to Les Gallo-Silver, senior social worker at New York

University Medical Center, the emotionally laden issues of fertility and sexual function are often viewed differently by men and women.

ॐ While male survivors are certainly concerned if they can't have children, they are usually much more concerned if they can't have an erection. Women, however, tend to view infertility as the major loss. Of course, a great deal of this has to do with culture: it's considered part of the female's role for them to bear children and for men to be strong and virile. This deeply ingrained societal message is difficult to ignore and can exert a lot of underlying emotional stress for those who don't fall in line with it. But even though cancer may alter one's sexual functioning or fertility status, it cannot extinguish the sexual self, the deep need we all have for love, closeness, and contact. ॐ

Sex Postcancer

Throughout their long marriage, Ed and his wife, Gina, have enjoyed an active, satisfying sex life. Both well into their sixties, they remained, according to Ed, "as ardent as adolescents." Even the stress and strain of juggling dual careers and parental responsibilities did little to impede their sexual life. They presumed nothing ever would, until Ed learned he had prostate cancer.

ॐ I went to see my urologist about problems I'd been having with frequent urination at night, as well as a sharp pain in my groin. I'd had plenty of PSA (prostate specific antigen) exams before, and my levels were always at about four. So when my urologist came back with an eleven reading, he and I both knew it was biopsy time.

Of course, you always figure you can prepare yourself psychically while you're waiting for the results. Although I thought I'd done that, it still came as a mind-numbing shock. My urologist presented the various treatment options: surgery, seed implant, radiation, chemotherapy, or "wait and watch." Then he ran down the side effects of each, explaining that with the radical prostatectomy there was a significant chance of permanent incontinence and that my sex life would be over. Maybe he said it differently than that, but that's what I heard.

It hit me hard, as I'm sure it hits all men. I've seen how deeply depressed some prostate cancer patients become over their problems with sexual dysfunction. It's the fear of that possibility that keeps too many men from going for prostate exams.

The doctor assured me that I didn't have to make an immediate decision, so Gina and I took a vacation to Alaska. Back home, we spent a great deal of time exploring the options, gathering information, and getting second opinions. Three months later, I decided on the surgery.

Not long after the prostatectomy, I did indeed begin having sexual problems. My urologist prescribed Viagra, but that didn't help. I was shown how to give myself injections directly into the side of my penis (intracorporeal injection), which provided me with a partial erection. But since the injections take about an hour to have an effect, the lack of spontaneity didn't work for me. My doc tried talking me into some sort of pump implant, but I wasn't comfortable with that idea either, so I passed.

I wasn't too happy about the long-term impact this was going to have on my wife. Even though our marriage is well established, and sex was only a part of it, a profound sense of guilt plagued me. We all know that sex isn't everything, but we live in an age when everyone acts like it is, so it's hard to buck those feelings. But Gina wouldn't have any of that kind of thinking, and instead reminds me daily that what is most important to her is that I'm still here. &

Like all newly diagnosed cancer patients, Ed's first thoughts were of survival. And like most patients, Ed chose the treatment option that would, in the experts' opinion, provide the best shot at securing long-term remission. But once the physical scars have healed and daily life reverts back to old routines, each of us is faced with the inevitable reckoning of the cost of survival and the impact it has on the quality of our lives.

After a radical prostatectomy, most males experience partial or total loss of the ability to achieve erection. For a certain percentage, partial sexual functioning may return gradually. For others, alternative treatment options, ranging from oral medications to penile prosthesis, can help insure a return of sexual functioning. However, as sex therapists explain, a gratifying sex life is more directly linked to an entirely different organ: the brain. Powerful emotions, about yourself as well as those close to you, have everything to do with how you reorient yourself back to sexual life. (If indeed it is an issue.) Body image and self-esteem are intrinsic to sexuality. Survivors who suffer from self-doubt, shame, or guilt, who view themselves as "damaged goods" or as somehow less than lovable, will have a more difficult time returning to a sense of sexual wellness.

Although frank talk about sexuality seems to be everywhere, when it comes to the touchy subject of sex after cancer, a great many people run for cover. It's a difficult topic for them to acknowledge and an awkward one to discuss. Older survivors, in particular, find it easier to closet the issue of altered sexuality or sexual dysfunction; some simply opt for celibacy.

Leslie Schover, Ph.D., author of the invaluable guide *Sexuality and Fertility After Cancer*, suggests that survivors be aware of the following situations — they may signal that it's necessary to seek professional help:

- Indefinitely putting off attempts at resuming sexual relations with a partner because of performance anxiety or lack of self-esteem.

- Avoiding social situations and dates because of negative perceptions about oneself.

- Feelings of unabated guilt, depression, anger, or grief over lost or diminished sexual functioning.

Schover stresses that with counseling and/or medical intervention, most sexual problems are surmountable. For survivors like Ed, the road back to a satisfying sex life begins with acknowledgment and acceptance. No one can guarantee that this will be an easy or speedy process. At the very least, it will require that you be open and honest about your feelings, in addition to remaining flexible to the kind of sexual adjustments that may be necessary to reestablish an active, satisfying sex life. In fact, Ed and many other survivors have discovered that the love and intimacy of a cherished relationship can actually grow and be made stronger as a result of their cancer.

The Loss of Fertility

Because cancer alters the view we have of ourselves, it frequently alters our vision of the future as well, a vision that for many of us includes having children. Survivors who are able to reproduce and choose to do so rarely enter into the decision lightly. Some hesitate, apprehensive that the physical and emotional demands of parenthood will prove too stressful, while others worry that the toxicity of cancer treatment may result in birth defects or an increased susceptibility to cancer in their offspring. Of greater concern to many survivors is the fear of a recurrence of the disease, and the significant burden that a seriously ill parent would be to a child.

Female survivors face additional concerns. Because certain chemotherapy drugs can damage the nervous system or weaken major internal organs such as the heart, lungs, or kidneys, women face the possibility of serious complications during pregnancy. Breast cancer survivors harbor an additional fear: that the surge of pregnancy-related hormones could stimulate a recurrence.

For some of us, these issues are moot. But for survivors like myself, the double blow of cancer *and* infertility can be overwhelming, or at the very least color one's outlook on dating, marriage, and parenthood. The loss of fertility is yet another reminder of how cancer has betrayed what we'd assumed was our right to a "normal" life; it is an additional insult to the self in terms of what it means to be like everyone else. Several Cancervive members have even told me that infertility presented a much larger crisis in their lives than cancer ever did. Ms. Michael Hubner, a social worker and project manager at Boston's Beth Israel Deaconess Medical Center, explains why:

⅋ Some recovered cancer patients find that coming to terms with infertility or altered sexuality means coming to terms with their cancer experience all over again and reliving that deep sense of loss and grief. It reminds them of their vulnerability and may revive long dormant and unresolved emotions.

This is particularly true of survivors of childhood cancer, many of whom were never told that treatment might result in reproduction problems. When they do learn of their treatment-induced infertility, it causes a crisis in their lives. ⅋

Of course, not every survivor faces the prospect of permanent sterility. And for some, the inability to have children is not a major concern. How a survivor will react to news of iatrogenic, or treatment-caused, infertility largely depends on the age as well as the life plan of that person. But if you're reading this chapter, chances are treatment-induced infertility is a concern in your life, and quite possibly a major one.

It certainly was for Kevin and Talia, two Cancervive members who triumphed over cancer only to learn that their victory had exacted the bitter compromise of infertility.

Kevin's Story

When Kevin was diagnosed with testicular cancer twenty years ago, he never gave much thought to how it might affect him later in life. Although he was informed that the disease and its treatment would likely result in sterility, Kevin, now forty-eight, and his wife weren't overly concerned. Like any couple facing a cancer diagnosis, they focused solely on the immediate crisis looming before them:

⅋ At the time of my diagnosis, my wife, Samantha, and I were in our twenties. The idea of having kids was still an abstract concept. But later, as our marriage began to unravel, I realized how shortsighted we'd been.

My cancer was a seminoma, a form of testicular cancer, possibly the result of an undescended testicle which had never been corrected. The surgeon excised it along with some lymph nodes and then, once that had healed, I was given radiation treatments. My medical team assured me that my prognosis was excellent, so my only real concern was getting through treatment.

Before the operation it was suggested that I look into sperm banking, and I'm glad I did. When I think about it now, that was really such a fateful decision, and yet I almost blew it off. Both Sam and I were struggling to make ends meet, and at the time the issue of kids was easier left undiscussed and undecided.

Tests at the sperm bank revealed that my sperm sample was low. My doctor advised me to go ahead and make a deposit anyway. And I did, even though I didn't see much point in it.

As it turned out, my treatment did result in sterility. At first, neither Sam nor I wanted to talk about it. It was like, "Hey, I can't complain. I survived cancer!" So once I'd bounced back, it was easier for both of us to simply shelve the issue and throw ourselves into work. But as time went on, it was hard for my wife to hide her resentment, and for me, my frustration and guilt. In addition, I was feeling insecure about my masculinity. My libido had taken a dive post-treatment, and I also had some problems with nerve damage and ejaculatory ability. Sam was more concerned about the fact that I was shooting blanks. Although I could handle a future without kids, she couldn't.

During one of my checkups, my doctor suggested we try having a baby through artificial insemination, using the sperm sample I'd banked. Sam went through all the tests and procedures and, to make a long story short, we spent a lot of time at the infertility clinic trying to make a go of it. But we weren't having much luck; my sperm sample wasn't up to speed.

The enormous anxiety and stress we were going through was putting a lot of strain on our relationship. We went into couples therapy, and that helped. But inevitably, the fact that I couldn't father kids always took center stage when we fought. We considered adopting a baby, but the adoption process intimidated me, and Sam wasn't wild about it either. We were close to calling it quits when Sam said she wanted to see another infertility specialist she'd heard about and give it one more try.

This time, she underwent in vitro fertilization, using my sperm sample and a process known as Intracytoplasmic Sperm Injection. When we saw the doctor for follow-up, we fully expected the thumbs-down verdict. Instead, we were stunned by the good news, not to mention wildly excited. Nevertheless, I continued to worry all through my wife's pregnancy, fearful that there might be a problem with fetal development because of the treatment I'd received. Happily, those fears were unfounded. That's not to say I don't worry about my daughter anymore. After all, she's now a teenager. ₧

Cancer's Effect on Male Fertility

As Kevin and Sam learned, coming to terms with the issue of sterility, fresh on the heels of a crisis with cancer, is a disruptive and difficult task. Left unresolved, the volatile emotions accompanying altered sexuality and infertility — anger, resentment, guilt, depression — inevitably interfere with a couple's feelings about intimacy and sexual activity.

Testicular cancer is the most common solid organ tumor diagnosed in men aged eighteen to thirty-five. When Kevin was diagnosed, oncologists were just beginning to understand how to successfully treat it. At the time, survival was by no means a sure thing. Today, the survival rate for this form of malignancy is more than 90 percent.

Unfortunately, the likelihood that treatment will result in sterility is also high. Studies reveal that following the acute stage of treatment, the majority of testicular cancer survivors will experience azoospermia, or absence of sperm, following treatment. Of these, approximately 60 percent will recover a normal sperm count after two or more years. Certain forms of radical surgery to a man's pelvic or abdominal area can damage pelvic nerves and lymphatics, which may cause problems with sexual functioning. During Kevin's surgery for testicular cancer, his doctors removed several lymph nodes from the surrounding pelvic area so that they could determine if his cancer had spread. This procedure, called retroperitoneal lymph node dissection, can disrupt sensitive nerve connections, which may in turn lead to a reduced ability to ejaculate. Surgery for colon cancer (colostomy), prostate cancer (prostatectomy), and bladder cancer (radical cystectomy) can also cause nerve damage to the penis, resulting in impaired fertility or altered sexual functioning.

The extent to which radiotherapy will affect a man's fertility depends primarily on the location of treatment and the total radiation dose. In many cases, men who receive radiation to the abdominal or pelvic area will experience either partial or full recovery of sperm production. But for some men, especially those who receive high-dose radiation to the gonads, infertility is often permanent.

In both males and females, due to the high-dose treatment involved, infertility and sterility are largely irreversible complications of bone marrow transplantation. Radiation treatment that results in permanent damage to the pituitary gland may also trigger sterility. Located at the base of the brain, the pituitary gland is often referred to as the "master gland" because it directs the body's hormonal output, including those hormones that stimulate sperm production (in males) and egg maturation (in females). As a result, sufficient irradiation to a patient's head may cause the pituitary gland to function abnormally, which in turn will throw hormonal production out of whack.

Because of the toxic nature of some anticancer drugs, chemotherapy can interfere with both male fertility and sexual functioning, although in most instances these problems will disappear soon after treatment. But the effect of chemotherapy is not uniform. Its impact on fertility depends on the class and dose of the drugs as well as the age of the patient. Survivors who received chemotherapy for bone sarcomas, Hodgkin's disease, non-Hodgkin's lymphoma, and leukemia are most at risk for permanent damage to their reproductive organs. A class of chemotherapy drugs known as alkylating agents appears to be the main culprit in chemo-related sterility. Among these, the commonly used drug cyclophosphamide (Cytoxan) is perhaps the most notorious. Other drugs known to suppress fertility are chlorambucil (Leukeran), bulsulfan (Myleran), and vinblastine (Velban).

Male survivors who suspect that treatment has caused problems with their fertility can ask their doctors to provide them with two simple tests: a semen analysis and a blood test. Through semen analysis, the physician can determine sperm count and motility as well as other factors that can interfere with fertility. A blood hormone test will detect the levels of essential male hormones in the body, including testosterone, follicle-stimulating hormone (FSH), and luteinizing hormone (LH). Every man needs sufficient levels of all three hormones for sperm production to take place.

A reminder to male survivors: although chemotherapy or radiation may have diminished or interrupted your sperm count or motility, this does not necessarily mean that you are unable to father children. In other words, don't rely on the effects of treatment as a method of birth control, especially if you are currently undergoing radiation or chemotherapy. If you have recently finished chemotherapy, your doctor may advise you or your partner to continue using some form of contraception since the effects of treatment on the reproductive system may linger for a year or more.

Semen Cryopreservation and Sperm-Banking

Semen cryopreservation, the technique Kevin used to bank his sperm, is particularly important to the male survivor whose initial cancer treatment was limited to surgery, but who may require future chemotherapy or radiation treatment. Kevin and Sam were able to conceive using Intracytoplasmic Sperm Injection (ICSI), a relatively new micromanipulation technique in which a single sperm is injected into an egg. Other assisted reproductive techniques include Gamete Intrafallopian Transfer (GIFT), or in vitro fertilization (IVF).

Success using these latter techniques is by no means guaranteed; IVF and GIFT carry a success rate of approximately 20 to 30 percent; with ICSI, the rate of fertilization is currently at about 65 percent.

The low sperm count that Kevin experienced is a condition that is often caused by the onset of cancer. This little-understood phenomenon is called subfertility and indicates a reduction in either the concentration or the motility of sperm. Doctors speculate that it may be one of the early effects cancer has on the body, perhaps a consequence of the disease's ability to depress levels of the hormones needed for proper functioning of the reproductive system.

Your oncologist or primary care physician can arrange to have you tested to determine if you are a good candidate for semen cryopreservation. At one time, subfertility posed a problem to men who chose to bank sperm. However, thanks to recent advances in male infertility technology, sperm-banking is highly recommended even when poor sperm motility or low sperm count are of concern. Like Kevin, many men have successfully fathered children from subfertile sperm samples utilizing the ICSI procedure.

The cost of sperm-banking is not an unreasonable concern. Frozen sperm samples remain viable for up to fifty years, and the cost of banking and maintenance is approximately $1,200 every five years. Check with your insurance company regarding coverage. To obtain more information about sperm banks and their locations in North America, contact the American Society for Reproductive Medicine at (205) 978-5000 or visit their Web site at www.asrm.com.

Talia's Story

It's one thing to be warned at the time of diagnosis that cancer treatment will impair your fertility, but quite another to find out years later, on your own. When twenty-two-year-old Talia came to her first Cancervive meeting more than a year ago, the issue of infertility was foremost in her mind. Like many young adults, Talia wasn't sure what she wanted out of the future. But she was sure of one thing: she wanted children.

When Talia was diagnosed with Hodgkin's disease at sixteen, she had no idea that treatment might affect her ability to fulfill that dream. Her parents were informed, but they held back on telling their daughter. Instead they decided to wait until after her recovery to break the news. But that time never came, and Talia was left to figure it out for herself.

&? I was treated with the MOPP [Mustargen, Oncovin, procarbazine, and prednisone] regimen of chemotherapy along with radiation. I bounced back pretty fast from it all, although my periods stopped shortly after my last treatment. At the time I didn't give it much thought since my doctor had warned me that chemotherapy would probably cause some irregularity. I actually enjoyed having a break from my monthly periods. But I wasn't expecting it to be permanent. More than a year later, I still wasn't menstruating, so I went to see a gynecologist. He was the first person to lay it on the line: my treatment had resulted in complete ovarian dysfunction. In other words, it was unlikely I'd ever have kids.

I left the office determined to get another opinion. Neither my oncologist nor my parents had ever told me that this would happen, so why should I believe this gynecologist? But as I drove home, everything he said began to sink in. By the time I got home, I was in tears and full of anger. That night I really ripped into my parents, yelling and screaming and accusing them. My mom just sat there crying. My dad tried to explain, saying that they had wanted to tell me, but felt that I'd handle it better when I was older. The way I see it, holding back that kind of information just made it worse.

I haven't had an easy time adjusting to the loss. It serves as another reminder of cancer, and that I'm somehow not normal because of it. Also, there's something so life-affirming about having a child. I've lost that, which I saw as a big part of my future, and now I've got to learn to make do. Sometimes I think I would have rather given up an arm or a leg in exchange for functioning ovaries. That's how strongly I feel about it.

The issue really complicates dating. It's a major hassle trying to tell a guy about all these things going on with me. When I do meet a guy I like, I feel that we have these invisible hurdles to cross before I can even think of a relationship with him. First, I have to find a way to tell him I had cancer. I prefer waiting until after we've had a few dates, so we have a chance to get to know one another. And I always put off having sex until after I've told him, otherwise it just complicates it too much for me emotionally. Once I've told him about the cancer — if he's still around — I'll go on to let him know that treatment caused me to be infertile. Then I brace for the reaction.

If nothing else, I've found this to be a great way of weeding out jerks. It's like, do I want to spend a lot of time with someone who can't accept me for who I am now? That's really what it all comes down to, you know? &·

Cancer's Effect on Female Fertility

In addition to learning that she was infertile, Talia carried the burden of a profound sense of anger and blame directed at her parents. Their solicitous attempts at protecting her by withholding news of her infertility backfired, seriously complicating her efforts at reconciling herself to her infertility. Les Gallo-Silver of New York University Medical Center explains why this happens with so many survivors of childhood cancer: "Balancing treatment options with fertility issues is an agonizing situation for every parent of a newly diagnosed child. When treatment does result in infertility, denial often becomes the knee-jerk reaction. After all, talking to your child about fertility entails recognizing your child as a sexual being, and many parents are simply too uncomfortable or embarrassed to tackle the subject. Other parents are so crushed by the stress and guilt of seeing their child endure cancer treatment that they don't want to be the bearers of more bad news. They hope that when they do finally have to face the infertility issue, their child will be more understanding and less likely to resent them for allowing it to happen."

Like Talia, many young women who receive chemotherapy won't suspect that they may have fertility problems until they are alerted to it by irregular menstrual cycles, which may or may not indicate the onset of premature menopause.

In many ways, a woman's reproductive life is much more complex than that of her male counterpart. A man's testicles perform the function of a twenty-four-hour semen factory, constantly producing new shipments of sperm. A woman, however, is born with a large but finite number of eggs (ova) in her ovaries, and that supply is slowly depleted throughout her reproductive life. Also, a woman's fertility is closely tied to her monthly menstrual cycle and the intricate hormonal commands that orchestrate it. Each month during ovulation, normally a single ovum is released from an ovary and begins its descent down the fallopian tubes toward the uterus. It is during this journey that the egg is poised for a potential rendezvous with sperm, and possible fertilization.

It doesn't take much to disrupt the precise synchronization of a woman's reproductive cycle, and cancer treatment can deliver a powerful shock to the system. Chemotherapy will do this by interfering with a woman's hormone production, which in turn interrupts the menstrual cycle, resulting in amenorrhea (suppressed menstrual period) or premature menopause. Cyclophosphamide (Cytoxan), mechlorethamine (Mustargen), chlorambucil (Leukeran), bulsulfan (Myleran), and vinblastine (Velban) are several chemo drugs known to interfere with ovarian function and menstruation. In most cases, this side effect reverses itself once treatment is complete. Whether these drugs cause permanent infertility or not usually depends on the dose involved and the length of therapy. The more aggressive and long-term chemotherapy is, the more likely a woman is to experience fertility problems.

Age also determines how well a woman's reproductive system endures treatment. For example, women aged twenty-five and under who undergo chemotherapy treatment involving the drug

Cytoxan will, in most cases, eventually experience a return of their normal menstrual cycle, whereas women who are in their thirties and early forties have a much greater chance of early menopause and permanent sterility.

Author and infertility expert Dr. Leslie Schover explains why age plays such an integral part in chemotherapy's effect on a woman's ovaries.

& A woman is born with all the eggs she'll ever have. Every month fifty or so of those eggs starts to mature, although usually only one makes it to full maturity. Reproductive endocrinologists use the term "ovarian reserve" to describe how many viable eggs remain in a woman's ovaries. The older you get, the more that reserve is used up. Chemotherapy destroys the follicles that nurture the eggs. In addition, it interferes with the hormone production of the ovaries. Younger women have greater ovarian reserve and may therefore have more capacity to recover from its effects. &

Schover adds that radiotherapy can also damage a woman's reproductive capacity, although the extent of that risk depends on the total dose and location of radiation as well as the age of the patient. For instance, radiation to a woman's pelvic area may interfere with her ability to have children if her treatment results in either ovarian failure or scarring of the vagina, uterus, or fallopian tubes. Women who are at greatest risk for permanent infertility are those who receive full radiation to the pelvic area in conjunction with chemotherapy.

New and innovative approaches to protect a patient's ovaries prior to treatment are constantly evolving. A recent approach employs the administration of briefer regimens of adjutant chemotherapy. Experimental studies also suggest that, for some patients, the ovaries can be protected during chemotherapy through the use of medication that temporarily halts ovulation. And in a method similar to sperm-banking, a technique known as ova retrieval allows women to freeze and store their eggs before they begin treatment. The frozen eggs may be fertilized at a later date and implanted in the woman's uterus.

Fertility may also be spared through the use of a technique known as ovarian transposition, which allows doctors to surgically block or relocate a woman's ovaries prior to radiation therapy. By this method, the surgeon physically moves the ovaries, complete with their blood supply, outside of the area that is going to be irradiated. This doesn't prevent the ovaries from functioning properly, but simply shields them from exposure. When radiation treatment is complete, the ovaries are then returned to their normal position. But the use of this procedure is relevant only to a small group of female cancer patients and depends primarily on the type of cancer and how near the ovaries the radiation will be delivered.

Oncologists continue to advance newer treatment techniques to further insure against the potential loss of a woman's childbearing ability, although options remain limited by the type of cancer and the scope of the treatment. If you are faced with treatment that may affect your fertility, talk to your medical team and express whatever concerns you have. Find out what treatment options are open to you and what, if anything, your doctors can do to diminish damage to your reproductive system.

Testing for Infertility

Many women assume that since cancer treatment has interrupted their periods, they must be infertile. The fact that you aren't menstruating, however, doesn't mean you can't get pregnant. (And, needless to say, a woman undergoing cancer treatment should not try to become pregnant during or immediately after treatment.) If your period was interrupted by the effects of treatment, your doctor probably won't be able to tell you when or if it will return. However, there are several tests you can take to find out your fertility status. These tests include:

- *Estradiol level test.* Estradiol is the most important of the estrogen hormones (female sex hormones) and can be used to measure the level of estrogen in your body. If treatment has resulted in total ovarian failure, estrogen will not be present in the bloodstream.

- *Serum FSH or LH test.* This test provides a more accurate indicator of ovarian dysfunction by measuring the amount of FSH (follicle stimulating hormone) and LH (luteinizing hormone) in the bloodstream. If these hormone levels are elevated, it can be a sign that both hormones are trying, albeit unsuccessfully, to stimulate ovulation.

- *Ovarian biopsy.* As a last resort, a doctor can perform this procedure to determine if you have any viable eggs left in your ovaries. The biopsy is performed surgically using a laparoscope to remove a tiny sample from the outer layer of an ovary. By studying this sample, your doctor can determine whether or not cancer treatment has actually destroyed all the eggs, resulting in complete ovarian failure. The procedure is painless and can be performed on an outpatient basis.

It is important to remember that for many women infertility is a temporary problem, even though it may take years to reverse itself. Unfortunately, doctors have no way of knowing which people will experience a reversal; for some, it just never happens. However, these tests will determine the status of your reproductive system.

Options to Infertility

Should preliminary tests reveal that you are either infertile or subfertile or that treatment-related problems have made it impossible for you to carry a baby to term, don't give up hope. Astonishing advances in medical technology are enabling many more infertile people to have a biological child through such assisted reproductive techniques as in vitro fertilization and embryo transfer. But as sophisticated as these procedures are, they don't work for everyone.

For some survivors, these options will ultimately prove to be too costly, inappropriate, or unsuccessful, in which case they may consider adoption.

However, should you opt to try for a biological child of your own, be sure to consult your gynecologist to help you decide which, if any, of the following assisted reproductive techniques might work for you.

Artificial Insemination by Husband (AIH)

Men who have either banked their sperm prior to treatment or who are experiencing subfertility as a result of their treatment can benefit from this procedure. With AIH, a man's sperm sample is deposited inside the woman's uterus at a time when she is known to be ovulating. Before performing this procedure, the doctor may medically process or "wash" the sperm sample to achieve better sperm concentration.

Artificial Insemination by Donor (AID)

In instances where the man is infertile and has no viable sperm sample, his mate may wish to undergo artificial insemination using sperm from an anonymous donor. The decision to use this method of conception is a highly personal one since the resulting embryo will not be biologically related to the father.

Since the outbreak of acquired immune deficiency syndrome (AIDS), infertile couples have voiced concern over the safety of donated sperm. You should know that sperm banks take stringent precautions to screen donor sperm for both genetic and sexually transmitted diseases. The American Fertility Society now recommends close monitoring and repeated testing of donor sperm for AIDS antibodies.

In Vitro Fertilization (IVF)

IVF (also known as artificial insemination) is an option for women with an intact uterus and one or two functioning ovaries. In vitro fertilization no longer inhabits the brave new world of reproductive medicine; it is now, in fact, standard medical practice. In this procedure, eggs are removed from a woman's ovaries and combined with a male's sperm sample in a laboratory dish. (In the early days of IVF, doctors used test tubes; hence the term "test-tube babies.") If fertilization occurs, the resulting pre-embryo is returned within a day or two to the woman's uterus.

In theory, IVF sounds relatively simple. In reality, it requires a great deal of patience and motivation as well as a considerable financial commitment by the couple, as do all assisted reproductive techniques. Subfertile men may benefit from IVF because fewer sperm are needed to fertilize the egg (although ICSI is now considered more effective). Even under auspicious laboratory conditions, however, fertilization may not occur if the sperm are abnormal or defective. Also, the woman's uterus must be functioning normally for the fertilized egg to implant successfully. Women who have experienced complete ovarian failure or removal of both ovaries may choose to try IVF using donor eggs.

Gamete Intrafallopian Transfer (GIFT), Zygote Intrafallopian Transfer (ZIFT), and Tubal Ovum Transfer

GIFT and ZIFT are both variations of the IVF procedure. With GIFT, several ripened eggs are harvested from the woman's ovaries, quickly mixed with sperm in a catheter, and then immediately transferred back into the woman's fallopian tube. (Both GIFT and ZIFT require that the woman have at least one healthy fallopian tube.) If fertilization occurs, the rapidly dividing pre-embryo will then travel down the fallopian tube to the uterus, where it may attach to the uterine lining. Because fertilization takes place within the woman's fallopian tubes, the GIFT procedure may come closest to duplicating natural conception.

In yet another variation known as zygote intrafallopian transfer, egg and sperm are first allowed to complete fertilization in a lab dish, and then the resulting pre-embryo (zygote) is placed back into the woman's fallopian tube. Candidates for either GIFT or ZIFT include the partners of men with low sperm counts and infertile women who choose to use donor eggs. Women in whom both fallopian tubes are blocked or those with damaged uteruses would not benefit from either of these procedures.

But there is hope for them. In a newer procedure known as tubal ovum transfer, the woman's eggs are surgically moved to the farthest end of one of her fallopian tubes, close to where it opens into the uterus. The egg is then fertilized through either intercourse or artificial insemination. Since this method allows the egg to be positioned beyond any part of either fallopian tube that may be damaged or blocked, it can be used when GIFT or ZIFT is not appropriate.

Ovum Donation (Donor Eggs)

What happens when cancer treatment causes a woman's ovaries to shut down permanently so that egg production and ovulation have ceased? Women who have been thrust by treatment into premature menopause have the option of using eggs donated by a close friend or relative. The donated egg is combined with the sperm of the infertile woman's partner and then transferred to her uterus or fallopian tubes. Before the transfer is made, doctors use hormone therapy to prepare the woman's uterus so that it will be receptive to the transplanted pre-embryo.

A major drawback to this method is the availability and cost of donor eggs. Not every infertile woman has a relative or friend who is willing to donate her genetic material. The issue then becomes whether or not to use eggs from an anonymous donor.

Before considering this option, you and your partner must ask yourselves what it will mean to raise a child who will be biologically related to only one of you. Should the child be given all the facts surrounding his or her conception, and if so, when? If a donor is used, will that person have a legal and financial responsibility to the child? And can you accept having a child through a procedure that is not yet considered socially secure? As you can see, there are a multitude of ethical and legal issues to address before considering this option.

Surrogacy

Hysterectomies and other forms of radical surgery to a woman's reproductive system almost always guarantee sterility. Women who have had hysterectomies can nevertheless still fulfill their hope of a biological child by "borrowing" another woman's uterus, most often that of either a friend or relative. The use of a paid surrogate is yet another, albeit controversial, option.

Two types of surrogacy exist. The first involves removing eggs from the sterile woman, provided of course that her ovaries are intact and producing healthy eggs. Her eggs are fertilized with her partner's sperm and the resulting pre-embryo is then transferred to the surrogate mother's uterus. If the procedure is successful, the surrogate will carry the infertile couple's baby to term.

In another form of surrogacy, the surrogate's own eggs are artificially inseminated with the sperm of the husband or mate of the infertile woman. The surrogate then surrenders the baby to the infertile couple at birth.

Surrogacy, like ovum donation, is an extraordinarily expensive, complex, and contentious issue, and survivors considering it need to carefully examine the legal and ethical ramifications involved.

Will you find success with any of these methods? It depends on a variety of factors, including your age and overall health, the cause of your infertility, and the quality of the sperm sample and its proficiency at fertilizing an egg. Should you decide to use a procedure that includes the biological participation of someone other than you and your mate (as with surrogacy, procedures using donor eggs, or AID), be sure to first consult a lawyer or social worker who is knowledgeable about the legal issues involved. You and your partner also need to weigh the emotional issues attached to these methods and discuss how your feelings will affect your relationship now and in the future.

Also, understand that these techniques are expensive, time-consuming, and emotionally exhausting. In addition, virtually all of them have a low success rate. If you plan to go ahead with infertility treatment, bear in mind that these procedures offer hope to some, not guarantees for all.

The Challenge of Adoption

What can be done if all of these assisted reproductive technologies fail? Reconciling one's dream of having a biological child with the hard, cold medical facts of infertility is a difficult task. The job then is to reshape our expectations around a different notion of parenthood, one that may include thoughts of adoption.

Before you can even think of moving on to this "second choice," you'll need to come to terms with your loss of fertility and resolve the emotions that loss has engendered. For many infertile couples, adoption means fully acknowledging the idea that the infant they bring home will not be genetically related to either partner. It also means accepting the possibility that even this alternative to parenting may ultimately elude them. But for those who do succeed in adopting, the joy of finally having a child to call their own can be overwhelming and the rewards endless.

For survivors of cancer, however, the issue of adoption is a great deal more complicated. Because of their medical history, recovered patients run a higher than average risk of rejection by traditional adoption agencies. Social worker Michael Hubner of Boston's Beth

Israel Deaconess Medical Center comments on the hesitation infertile survivors feel when their thoughts turn to adoption:

&ペ For those who have already experienced cancer treatment and infertility, leaving themselves open to that kind of rejection and emotional loss all over again is even more devastating than it would be for the normal infertile person. You desperately want the chance to adopt a child, yet you want to spare yourself any further loss or injury to self-esteem. These conflicting desires can, in effect, paralyze a survivor's attempt at adoption. &ペ

The process of adopting through traditional agencies is often complex, anguishing, and fraught with frustration. As an alternative, many survivors turn to private adoption, in which the couple deal directly with the birth mother or through an intermediary such as a lawyer or doctor. But survivors and social workers have informed me that private adoption comes with its own unique pitfalls. For instance, private adoption tends to cost much more than traditional adoptions. Then again, like other infertile people, survivors run the risk of having the birth mother renege on her promise to surrender the baby.

Of course, not every survivor who chooses adoption faces certain rejection. The criteria that adoption agencies use to screen applicants vary widely from state to state, although the basic requirements are fairly standard. For example, adoption agencies consider only couples who are in "stable relationships" — that is, those who have been married for several years and who have what the agency regards as sound financial and social backgrounds. Most traditional agencies will not even consider divorced or single persons. Your date of birth also comes into play: agencies generally regard age forty as the limit for eligibility.

For survivors, however, the stumbling block to adoption lies in the medical history requirement. Many have found that the adoption process comes to a screeching halt once the word "cancer" is mentioned. Long-term survivors even say that they have a difficult time convincing either the agency or the birth mother that they are indeed disease-free, despite the fact that their physicians have confirmed it in writing.

What does this mean? Will the stigma associated with cancer demolish your chances? Infertility expert Dr. Leslie Schover responds:

&? Adoption, even for couples without preexisting medical conditions, is increasingly difficult, complex, and expensive. Many public adoption agencies simply won't disclose the criteria they use to choose parents. My concern is that given all the eligible couples that apply, they are likely to place the cancer survivor's name at the bottom of the list, regardless of how good that person's prognosis is. The same thinking applies to private adoptions, where the birth mother makes the decision. It would take a great deal of sophistication and empathy on the part of the birth mother to seriously consider someone with a history of cancer as the potential parent of their infant. &?

According to Schover, the most important signal a survivor can send to an adoption agency or birth mother is one of hope and confidence. But if unresolved emotions are still churning inside you, they may undermine your confidence and affect how you present yourself.

Then again, not every infertile person is eager to become a parent. Some survivors are content to remain child-free. For these people, life without children makes perfect sense; it fits their lifestyle and plans for the future. Contrary to what society tells us, children aren't necessarily a requisite for happiness and self-fulfillment. It all depends on your outlook. When feminist Gloria Steinem, herself a survivor of breast cancer, was asked why she decided not to have children, she replied, "I had a choice: I either gave birth to someone else or I gave birth to myself."

The Emotions of Infertility

How will you react when tests reveal that your infertility is irreversible? Even though you may have suspected it, your prognosis still comes as a palpable blow. Once you've absorbed this information, you may find initial feelings of shock melting into denial or anger. You know the reaction. You'll hear yourself saying, "This isn't happening to me!" For some people, the news is so painful that they protect themselves by rejecting it, or by pretending that their infertility is only a temporary problem.

According to family therapist Christine Perkins, denial plays an important part in allowing the mind to adjust slowly to the news of infertility.

❧ Like a psychic Band-Aid, denial can protect you during the time you are most vulnerable. But sooner or later you'll need to get past denial so that you can heal completely. Grieving will give you the opportunity to rework your self-image so that your sexuality and self-esteem are no longer so dependent on whether or not you can have children. ❧

Many survivors become trapped in the denial stage, however, unwilling or unable to relinquish their dream of having children. They choose to continue harboring the hope that one day they will confound the odds, surprise the doctors, and succeed in giving birth. As years go by and the reality of infertility sinks in, their denial may suddenly and unexpectedly give way to anger and resentment. Says Perkins, "Anger is an important part of the grieving process; it compels you to react to what you perceive to be the injustice of your infertility."

Like Kevin and Talia, you may find yourself projecting your anger onto those you believe to be most responsible: your parents, the oncologist, God, yourself. You may also find that getting beyond the blame and resentment isn't easy. Michael Hubner, of the Beth Israel Deaconess Medical Center, says that the anger survivors feel is much more complicated than the anger felt by other infertile people:

❧ It's a strange sort of blunted anger, because you're angry at the people who made the decision to save your life. It's not a clear-cut emotion, and certainly not easy to resolve. As a result, you may feel guilty over the way you are reacting. ❧

In addition, your anger may be a reaction to the loss of control that both cancer and infertility represent. As a survivor, you already live with a heightened sense of vulnerability, an unsettling realization that your body, once so self-sufficient and reliable, isn't always going to keep you safe or do your bidding.

Survivors often point out that infertility, like cancer, sets them apart; they often feel alienated from their peers, even from other infertile people. Like Talia, many single survivors who are infertile worry about dating and establishing close relationships. They see themselves as biological failures, outcasts from the gene pool, and therefore undesirable to the opposite sex.

In fact, some survivors become so sensitized to the issue of infertility that they avoid people and social events that may remind them of it. Talia says that for several years she had trouble socializing with girlfriends who were either pregnant or new mothers.

❧ I remember going to my best friend's baby shower two years after I'd learned about my infertility. I thought that I was beyond all the heavy emotions. But I felt so envious and angry at the shower that I left early and cried all the way home. Since then I've found it easier to stay away from baby showers and children's birthday parties. ❧

Reaching Out

The emotions of infertility are personal and complex as well as puzzling and painful. You may not be able to resolve your grief by

228 & Can Survive

yourself, and you shouldn't feel that you have to. Infertility is a life crisis shared by millions of people, some of them survivors. Because of the nature of cancer treatment, the National Cancer Institute estimates that infertility is 15 percent more common among survivors than among other adults. In short, you are not alone.

One important source of emotional support is Resolve, the national nonprofit organization for infertile people. This Massachusetts-based organization has been offering infertility counseling, referrals, and support to members since 1973. With the help and support of groups like Resolve and the healing powers of time and faith, many people have learned how to accept their infertile status. Call your local chapter of Resolve for information about group meetings or to learn about other Resolve members in your area who are also cancer survivors. Headquarters for Resolve are at 1310 Broadway, Somerville, MA 02144 (617-623-0744); Web site: www.resolve.org.

When all is said and done, infertility cannot change who you are. You still have the capacity to love, to create, to appreciate life, and to leave your mark on the world. It took me many years, as well as counseling and the support of loved ones, before I could fully accept my own infertility. Learn to let go of your loss and find ways to feel good about yourself. Cancer treatment may have taken away your ability to have children, but it has given you the gift of life and the prospect of a rewarding future. It's a bittersweet victory, but a victory nonetheless.

Paving the Way

In many ways, today's recovered cancer patients are like trailblazers, clearing a wilderness of survivorship issues, paving a path for others to follow. They are doing this by speaking up about such post-treatment complications as altered sexuality and infertility and expressing how these issues affect the quality of survival. They are clearing the way for future patients by drawing attention to patients' rights and demanding more informed consent. Doctors are in turn responding by providing additional information, seeking less toxic therapies, and doing what they can to minimize reproductive damage. But, as Michael Hubner of Beth Israel Deaconess Medical Center notes, much more needs to be done:

🚲 Even though cancer survival rates have improved, there is still no vocal constituency of young survivors who are speaking up and telling the medical community, "Look at us. We are surviving five, ten, even thirty years or more after diagnosis. And infertility is one of the many issues we continue to confront." Like other advocacy groups, cancer survivors must organize the effort and demand change. They need to focus attention on the issue of infertility and continue to raise the consciousness of health care providers by asking "Why wasn't I told?" and "Why aren't there any real alternatives?" 🚲

This message came across loud and clear when, at a recent Cancervive meeting, a member noted, "When you think about it, we're all part of a transitional generation. Fifty years ago, none of us would have been lucky enough to be here, talking about infertility."

Talia was at that meeting. She replied by saying, "But you know what? In ten years there will be another group of people sitting here who will have survived cancer with their fertility intact. And it will be, in no small part, because of people like us."

10

Cancervive: Acceptance and Advocacy

> "I will act as if what I do makes a difference."
> — William James

THIS BOOK BEGAN with a journey. It is only fitting that it should end with a look at where that journey has led and the discoveries I made along the way.

Following our initial support group meeting in 1985, my co-founder Lisa and I realized how much the burgeoning survivor population needed an organization like Cancervive. It filled a void in cancer care previously overlooked by the medical community.

Galvanized by our emotional commitment, we had plunged headlong into fulfilling our dream without really knowing how to make it a working reality. After all, how did one go about setting up a nonprofit organization? What kind of programs should we offer? How would we raise the funds to support our activities?

"We just *do* it," said Lisa matter-of-factly when I called her in San Francisco to report the success of the first few meetings. "We'll do what we can and we'll ask for help when we need it. And I promise, as soon as I can escape from this hospital, I'll be there to give you a hand."

Lisa's enthusiasm and desire to help belied her physical condition; the long-term complications of treatment were continuing to take their toll on her. The hospital was now her primary place of residence as she underwent innumerable medical procedures. Her input and participation in Cancervive became limited to talks on the phone from her hospital bed.

Lisa's plight spurred me on. Five hundred miles south in Los Angeles, I began putting together Cancervive's board of directors and organizing more support group meetings. With the financial and emotional support of my parents, I quit my job and dedicated myself full-time to our fledgling organization. I set up a makeshift office in my apartment and was on the phone every day with media people, hospital administrators, and oncology social workers.

Fundraising was, of course, a constant concern, and Lisa and I plotted ways of ferreting out financial support. Help would often appear unsolicited. An acquaintance offered to provide us with her services as a public relations consultant. A local firm donated a personal computer. A typesetting shop owned by a cancer survivor offered to prepare our newsletter free of charge. Small miracles like this assured me that Cancervive was going to thrive.

With the help of two social workers, I set down the organization's basic philosophy. We decided that a person must be considered disease-free and off treatment before joining a Cancervive support group. Initially, many people questioned my insistence on this point. They asked, "Isn't anyone with a cancer diagnosis essentially a survivor?" I didn't think so. In my view, the cancer patient and the survivor are at two distinctly different developmental stages. I knew this from my own experience, and the many health professionals I spoke to concurred with my view. As a survivor, my needs and concerns were centered around the challenges of life after cancer — issues related to the disease but as distinct from the patient stage as spring from winter.

I also wanted Cancervive to serve as a sort of lightship to guide recovered patients once they had navigated their way through treatment and were headed back into the mainstream. I remember taking a call from a woman who had recently been diagnosed with leukemia. She was interested in attending one of our support groups. I explained to her the criterion for joining Cancervive and then gave her a number of referrals to patient-oriented support groups. I hung up the phone feeling vaguely depressed, as if I'd somehow let her down. Two days later I received a large donation in the mail. To my surprise, it was from the woman with leukemia. Along with the check, she included a note: "This is to assure that Cancervive will be there for me once I become a survivor."

Within a few months, my two telephone lines were swamped with calls from people wanting to know more about the organization. Word spread about our support groups and the feedback from those who attended our meetings was phenomenal.

"It helps so much to hash out my problems with people who can identify with them," said one woman. Another person observed, "At other cancer support groups, I always felt that, as a survivor, I was supposed to serve as the 'example' to group members who were still fighting the disease. At Cancervive I don't have to worry about putting on a front." Someone else said simply, "I'm so relieved to know I'm not alone."

Lisa was delighted to hear about the groundswell of support Cancervive was receiving. "We've finally found our oasis in the desert!" she cheered. Our dream was now a tangible reality.

To my surprise, Cancervive was having a powerful effect on me as well. I had been so busy with the nuts and bolts of running a non-profit organization that I was slow to realize how my involvement in it was changing my life. I felt as if I'd finally reached a point where I could integrate my cancer experience into who I was and share what I'd learned in a positive way with other people.

Of course, that kind of self-acceptance didn't arrive overnight. Instead it was a gradual, evolutionary process. One particular incident sticks in my mind as the turning point. I was on a flight returning from Washington, D.C., where I had attended a conference on issues facing survivors. The flight was crowded, and I was exhausted. To make matters worse, my right leg was swollen and sore. I couldn't have been doing a very good job of hiding my discomfort because the man sitting next to me turned and asked if something was wrong. My first impulse was to discount my leg and pretend that I was fine. But something made me stop and think, Why should I lie? What do I have to hide? Instead, I told him that cancer treatment for my leg many years ago had resulted in a chronic swelling problem.

"You mean you have lymphedema?" he asked. "Wouldn't it help if you elevated it? Here, use my knee to prop up your leg."

I was pleasantly surprised by his openness and concern, and without hesitation took him up on the offer. As it turned out, he was married to a woman who also had lymphedema. He explained that his wife's condition was the result of a radical mastectomy. We talked about cancer, my organization, and the issues of survivorship all the way to Los Angeles. On that flight I made up my mind to "come clean" with my cancer history. I no longer felt the need to lie to strangers or cloak my disabled leg in alibis.

The layers of protection I'd used all those years to insulate myself began to fall away, and in the process my personal life grew more fulfilling. I know now that survivors need to make peace with what has happened to them. Until we learn to make the experience a positive and constructive force in our lives, our relationships will always be loaded down by the emotional baggage left over from cancer. That's certainly how it was for me.

One of my favorite poems, "Don't Ask," by the Chilean poet Pablo Neruda, alludes to a person who is forever lugging around a sack of stones. Each of us, in our own way, carries around a cache of stones. You either learn to be comfortable carrying around those stones, or you find a way to lay them aside. Survivors need a place to unburden themselves of fear, anger, and sadness. That, quite simply, is the reason for support groups like Cancervive.

In my view, that's also the significance of all support groups. They provide a safe haven, a collective atmosphere of caring and support to tell our stories, exchange insights, and gain information from the true experts: other people who have been there. Shared experience is the glue that forms an instant bond between members, a sort of comradeship of the campfire. In that sense, a support group can provide the kind of psychological salve that promotes healing. It is also an effective antidote to the isolation, the sense of aloneness, that is so much a part of cancer's terrain.

At a Cancervive support group meeting, I asked several members to discuss what they had gained from belonging to the group.

Jose Luis: Cancervive is different from any other support group I've attended. Other groups included people who were still in treatment. They were in the middle of that intense, fight-for-your-life stage. How could I talk about my problems as a survivor when in comparison my worries seemed so insignificant? But here I feel like I can be open about what's really bothering me.

Nora: As a survivor, I now find I have the emotional distance to make sense of what happened to me as a patient. Talking to other survivors helps me put it in perspective and distill from it all kinds of insights. It becomes a process of healing.

Jesse: I appreciate that Cancervive support groups don't meet in a hospital setting. My group meets in a hotel conference room, and for me, it's much more relaxing that way. There's something about meeting in a hospital that puts me in a "patient" state of mind, and I don't see myself in that role anymore. As it is, it's depressing enough having to go back to the hospital for checkups.

Lena: My marriage broke up several months after my treatment for melanoma. When I first came to the group I wasn't sure I would ever make sense of what had happened. To my surprise, I found myself crying in front of total strangers. They knew the kind of confusion and pain I was feeling in a way none of my friends could. This group has been my emotional anchor.

Tasha: Even though I have a very loving and supportive family, they can't really understand what I've gone through, and that's a lonely feeling. I imagine it's the way combat veterans feel when they come home from war, or survivors of airplane crashes. The experience has made you part of a special group, those who have "been there." You come away from it with a different view of life.

Anita: People always think that once treatment ends, a cancer patient's life magically falls back into place. But I think that's the rare exception. In many ways, being a survivor is much harder than being a patient. That's when the isolation sets in, and the fear of recurrence. A survivor support group is really a first-line defense against that.

Paul (*to Anita*): I know what you mean. But it wasn't easy for me to understand at first. It took me a while to accept that I might feel better talking about cancer. For me, it was the whole macho thing — grin and bear it. During my recovery, my family didn't want to hear about cancer anymore. And they certainly didn't want me talking about what might happen if I got a recurrence. I took their cue and started denying a lot of what I was really feeling. But fear of recurrence has been the big hurdle for me, and that was rough facing by myself. When it started getting the better of me, I decided I needed to do something. The first few support group meetings I went to I didn't say a word. Now they practically have to tell me to shut up.

Iris: That's just it! In a support group you can let it all hang out, really be yourself, not someone you think others want you to be. It's a safe place to raise issues you can't verbalize anywhere else. For instance, no one wants to hear me talk about being infertile. But at Cancervive, I can really open up about a lot of stuff that's bothering me without someone judging me.

Linda: One of the great things about a group like Cancervive is that I can learn from other people's coping techniques. When I found out that my chemo-related hearing problems would be permanent, I was angry. At a meeting, I heard Jose Luis mention that when he gets upset he shuts himself in a room and screams it out. That kind of therapy had never occurred to me before. I decided to try it. I got in my car one night, drove out to a deserted spot, turned the radio up high, and started screaming my lungs out. I kept it up until I was completely exhausted. And you know what? It really helped. The only trouble is that whenever I do it, I have to keep an eye out for the cops. It's embarrassing having to explain my "primal scream" therapy to them.

The reasons for joining a support group are as diverse as the individuals who attend them. But two common bonds unite these people: a history of cancer and the desire to talk about it with other survivors. Talk may be cheap, but don't overlook its curative powers. There's something wonderfully reassuring about hearing how fellow survivors have handled the dark demons of fear and anger, guilt and depression. Research now suggests that peer-to-peer support is good for your physical health as well. Physicians at Stanford University and the University of California–Berkeley have discovered that cancer patients who receive emotional and social support through group therapy tend to survive up to twice as long as patients who rely on medical treatment alone. Communication, it would seem, is not only therapeutic but life-giving as well.

At the heart of every survivor support group is a celebration of life, stripped of its materialistic trappings, pared down to an elegant understanding of what it means to be alive. A cancer diagnosis splashes you with a sort of ontological awareness, and survival hones that awareness into a steely-edged wisdom. People who have recovered from cancer savor life as only survivors can.

Of course, not everyone is comfortable being a "groupie" — and that's okay too. Some survivors have told me that they don't respond well to what they perceive as the "touchie-feelie" nature of support groups. Others say they have trouble coping with other people's problems; it compounds their own pain and suffering. Then again, some people just prefer to keep their emotions private. For these people there are always other options such as individual therapy, meditation, or prayer, to name just a few. Only you can know what approach works best for you.

But if you haven't visited a support group, I suggest you give it a try. Survivors who appear to gain the most from group therapy are individuals who have decided to accept cancer as part of their identity and are in search of ways to integrate the experience. Since starting Cancervive I've noticed that survivors often arrive at this decision at different times in their lives.

For instance, three years ago a young woman, a survivor of osteogenic sarcoma (bone cancer), came to her first Cancervive meeting. She said very little at the meeting, offering only that during her treatment doctors had performed a limb salvage procedure to save her leg. Afterward she approached me and inquired about my limp. I told her about my cancer treatment, its effect on my leg, and how I had dealt with the repercussions. We parted ways, and she never came back. I concluded that Cancervive simply didn't offer the kind of help she was looking for. But several months ago, that same woman resurfaced and has been attending meetings on a regular basis ever since. She admitted that seeing my disabled leg at that first meeting terrified her because doctors had told her that one day she might have trouble walking as a result of her treatment. Three years ago she hadn't been ready to accept that; now she was. I know that it wasn't easy for her to get to that point. More than a decade ago, I too began the same process of taking stock. And I learned that very often beginning the journey is as important as arriving at the destination.

Lisa and I started Cancervive with the hope that through our organization and others like it we could chip away at cancer's stubborn stigma and the barriers it creates. It is my desire that survivors will one day feel proud of having had cancer, and that others will come to regard it, in the words of Dr. Fitzhugh Mullan, as "a gritty badge of distinction." Lisa and I always felt that because of our cancer we had something special to offer the world — an alertness to life's nuances, a keener insight into others, a resiliency and strength that comes from having stared down death and faced up to the battle.

Lisa's own battle ended on August 14, 1988. During her final months in the hospital, she did her best to convince me that her condition wasn't as serious as it seemed. I used to say she had nine lives, but this time I knew I was losing her. If nothing else, I wanted Cancervive to stand for Lisa's long, brave struggle. To me, her courage, determination, and vitality exemplified what it means to be a survivor.

I never got the chance to say goodbye to Lisa, but there isn't a day that goes by that I don't feel her presence; it's there at every support group meeting. As difficult as it was coming to terms with her death, I found acceptance came in small steps, with each new achievement of the goals we had set. It remains no small comfort to think how proud she would be to know the positive effect Cancervive has had in the lives of so many people.

Surviving cancer is an experience wrought with pain, hope, anger, and laughter. The disease challenges our ability to endure. By sifting through our losses and gains, by accepting and letting go, we seek not just to endure but to thrive. And for survivors, that's the riskiest and noblest challenge of all.

Bibliography

Anders, George. *Health Against Wealth*. New York: Mariner, 1996.

Andrieu, Jean Marie, M.D., and Maria Elena Ochoa-Molina. "Menstrual Cycle, Pregnancies and Offspring Before and After MOPP Therapy for Hodgkin's Disease." *Cancer* 52 (1983): 435–39.

Bessier, Arnold R., M.D. "Denial and Affirmation in Illness and Health." *American Journal of Psychiatry* 136 (August 1979): 1026–30.

Boulad, Farid, M.D.; Sands, Stephen, Psy.D.; Sklar, Charles, M.D. "Late Complications after Bone Marrow Transplantation in Children and Adolescents." *Current Problems in Pediatrics* 28 (October 1998): 273–304.

Broyard, Anatole. "Doctor, Talk to Me." *New York Times Magazine*, August 25, 1990.

———. "Intoxicated by My Illness." *New York Times Magazine*, November 12, 1989.

Bruning, Nancy. *Coping with Chemotherapy*. New York: Doubleday, 1993.

Caroll-Johnson, Rose Mary, R.N., Linda M. Gorman, R.N., and Nancy Jo Bush, R.N., eds., *Psychosocial Nursing Care*. Pittsburgh: Oncology Nursing Press, 1998.

Cassileth, Barrie R., Ph.D., et al. *The Cancer Patient*. Ed. Barrie R. Cassileth, Ph.D. Philadelphia: Lea & Febiger, 1979.

Chesler, Mark A., and Oscar A. Barbarin. *Childhood Cancer and the Family*. New York: Brunner/Mazel, 1987.

Christ, Grace A. "Social Consequences of the Cancer Experience." *American Journal of Pediatric Hematology/Oncology* 9 (1987): 84–88.

Clark, Matt, with Holly Morris et al. "Learning to Survive." *Newsweek*, April 8, 1985.

Cousins, Norman. *Anatomy of an Illness*. New York: Norton, 1979.

———. *Head First*. New York: Dutton, 1989.

Crothers, Helen. "Health Insurance: Problems and Solutions for People with Cancer Histories." Paper presented at the American Cancer Society's

Proceedings of the Fifth National Conference on Human Values and Cancer, San Francisco, 1987: 100–109.

Dackman, Linda. *Up Front: Sex and the Post-Mastectomy Woman.* New York: Viking, 1990.

Davidsson, Glen W. *Understanding Mourning: A Guide for Those Who Grieve.* Minneapolis: Augsburg, 1984.

Dietz, J. Herbert, Jr., M.D. *Rehabilitation Oncology.* New York: Wiley, 1981.

Dobkin, Patricia, and Gary R. Morrow, Ph.D. "Long-Term Side Effects in Patients Who Have Been Successfully Treated for Cancer." *Journal of Psychosocial Oncology* 3 (Winter 1985/86): 23–51.

Dollinger, Malin, M.D., Ernest H. Rosenbaum, M.D., and Greg Cable. *Everyone's Guide to Cancer Therapy.* Missouri: Andrews McMeel Publishing, 1997.

Downie, Patricia A. *Cancer Rehabilitation.* London: Faber & Faber, 1976.

Enteen, Robert. *Health Insurance: How to Get It, Keep It, or Improve What You've Got.* New York: Demos Vermande, 1996.

Feldman, Frances L. "Wellness and Work." In *Psychosocial Stress and Cancer,* edited by C. L. Cooper. New York: Wiley, 1984.

Fiore, Neil A. *The Road Back to Health.* New York: Bantam, 1990.

Fishman, Steve. "Cancer Comes Home." *New York Times Magazine,* June 11, 1989.

Fromer, Margot Joan. *Surviving Childhood Cancer.* Washington, D.C.: American Psychiatric Press, Inc., 1995.

Gogan, Janis L., et al. "Pediatric Cancer Survival and Marriage: Issues Affecting Adult Adjustment." *American Journal of Orthopsychiatry* 49 (July 1979): 423–30.

Goldberg, Richard J., M.D., and Robert M. Tull, Ph.D. *The Psychosocial Dimensions of Cancer.* New York: Macmillan, 1983.

Goldenberg, S. Larry, M.D. *Intelligent Patient Guide to Prostate Cancer,* 2nd ed. Vancouver: Intelligent Patient Guide, Ltd., 1997.

Goodman, Ellen. *Turning Points.* New York: Fawcett Columbine, 1979.

Graham, Jory. *In the Company of Others.* New York: Harcourt Brace Jovanovich, 1982.

Grealy, Lucy. *Autobiography of a Face.* Boston: Houghton Mifflin, 1994.

Green, Daniel M., M.D. *Long-Term Complications of Therapy for Cancer in Childhood and Adolescence.* Baltimore: Johns Hopkins University Press, 1989.

Greenberg, Mimi, Ph.D. *Invisible Scars.* New York: Walker, 1988.

Greenhouse, Linda, "High Court Limits Who Is Protected by Disability Law." *New York Times,* June 23, 1999.

Hamilton, Joan O. C. "The Prognosis on Health Care: Critical — and Getting Worse." *Business Week,* January 9, 1989.

Hendin, Herbert, and Ann Pollinger Haas. *Wounds of War.* New York: Basic Books, 1984.

Holland, Jimmie C., Ph.D., and Julia H. Rowland, Ph.D., eds. *Handbook of Psycho-Oncology.* New York: Oxford University Press, 1998.

Johnson, Judi L., R.N., Ph.D., and Linda Klein. *I Can Cope: Staying Healthy with Cancer.* Minneapolis: DCI Publishing, 1994.

Kalter, Suzy. *Looking Up.* New York: McGraw-Hill, 1987.

Kauffman, Danette G. *Surviving Cancer.* Washington, D.C.: Acropolis, 1987.

Keene, Nancy. *Childhood Leukemia.* Sebastopol, CA: O'Reilly & Associates, Inc., 1997.

Kleinman, Arthur, M.D. *The Illness Narratives.* New York: Basic Books, 1988.

Koocher, Gerald P., Ph.D., and John E. O'Malley, M.D. *The Damocles Syndrome.* New York: McGraw-Hill, 1981.

Koocher, Gerald P., et al. "Psychological Adjustment Among Pediatric Cancer Survivors." *Journal of Child Psychology and Psychiatry* 21 (1980): 163–73.

Korda, Michael. *Man to Man.* New York: Random House, 1996.

Kübler-Ross, Elisabeth, M.D. *On Death and Dying.* New York: Macmillan, 1969.

Lacher, Mortimer J., M.D., and John R. Redman, M.D. *Hodgkin's Disease: The Consequences of Survival.* Philadelphia: Lea & Febiger, 1990.

LaMaistre, JoAnn, Ph.D. *After the Diagnosis.* Berkeley, Calif.: Ulysses Press, 1995.

Lansky, Shirley B., M.D., Marcy A. List, Ph.D., and Chris Ritter-Sterr, M.S. "Psychosocial Consequences of Cure." *Cancer* 58 (1986): 529–33.

Laufer, Robert S., M. S. Gallops, and Ellen Frey-Wouters. "War Stress and Trauma: The Vietnam Veteran Experience." *Journal of Health and Social Behavior* 25 (March 1984): 65–85.

Leerhsen, Charles, with Shawn D. Lewis et al. "Unite and Conquer." *Newsweek,* February 5, 1990.

Leporrier, Michel, M.D., et al. "A New Technique to Protect Ovarian Function Before Pelvic Irradiation." *Cancer* 60 (1987): 2201–4.

Lerner, Harriet Goldhor, Ph.D. *The Dance of Anger: A Woman's Guide to Changing the Patterns of Intimate Relationships.* New York: Harper & Row, 1986.

Lifton, Robert Jay. *Home from the War.* New York: Simon & Schuster, 1973.

Ludtke, Melissa. "Can the Mind Help Cure Disease?" *Time,* March 12, 1990.

Mathiessen, Constance. "Unsurance." *Hippocrates,* November/December 1989.

Meadows, Anna T., M.D., and Wendy L. Hobbie. "The Medical Consequences of Cure." *Cancer* 58 (1986): 524–28.

Menning, Barbara Eck. "The Infertile Couple: A Plea for Advocacy." *Child Welfare* 54 (June 1975): 454–60.

Monmaney, Terrence, and Eduardo Levy-Spira with Mary Hager. "Young Survivors in a Deadly War." *Newsweek,* July 18, 1988.

Morra, Marion, and Eve Potts. *Triumph: Getting Back to Normal When You Have Cancer.* New York: Avon, 1990.

Mullan, Fitzhugh, M.D. "The Cancer Consort: Making Cancer Survivors a Positive Political Force." *Journal of Psychosocial Oncology* 5 (Spring 1987): 81–87.

———. "Needed: An Agenda for Survivors." *Cope,* November 1986.

———. "Seasons of Survival: Reflections of a Physician with Cancer." *New England Journal of Medicine* 313 (1985): 270–73.

Nader, Ralph, and Wesley J. Smith. *Winning the Insurance Game.* New York: Knightsbridge, 1990.

Northouse, Laurel L. "Living with Cancer." *American Journal of Nursing* (May 1981): 961–62.

Parachini, Allan. "Cancer Survivors: Coping with Life." *Los Angeles Times,* September 1, 1985, sec. 6.

Patterson, James T. *The Dread Disease: Cancer and Modern American Culture.* Cambridge: Harvard University Press, 1987.

Podrasky, Patricia Anne. "The Family Perspective of the Cured Patient." *Cancer* 58 (1986): 522–23.

Redman, John R., et al. "Semen Cryopreservation and Artificial Insemination for Hodgkin's Disease." *Journal of Clinical Oncology* 5 (February 1987): 233–38.

Riekler, Patricia P., Susan D. Edbril, and Marc B. Garnick. "Curative Testis Cancer Therapy: Psychosocial Sequelae." *Journal of Clinical Oncology* 3 (August 1985): 1117–26.

Roberts, Leslie. *Cancer Today: Origins, Prevention, and Treatment.* Washington,
D.C.: National Academy Press, 1984.

Roemer, Ruth, M.D. "The Right to Health Care — Gains and Gaps."
American Journal of Public Health 78 (March 1988): 241–47.

Rosenthal, Elisabeth. "The Cancer War: A Major Advance." *New York Times
Magazine,* October 8, 1989.

Scarf, Maggie. *Intimate Partners: Patterns in Love and Marriage.* New York:
Random House, 1987.

Schover, Leslie R. *Sexuality and Fertility After Cancer.* New York: John
Wiley & Sons, 1997.

Segal, Julius, Ph.D. *Winning Life's Toughest Battles.* New York: Ivy Books, 1986.

Silberner, Joanne. "First, You Beat the Cancer." *U.S. News & World Report,*
November 6, 1989.

Simonton, Stephanie Matthews. *The Healing Family.* New York: Bantam,
1984.

Slaby, Andrew E., M.D. *Aftershock.* New York: Villard, 1989.

Smedes, Lewis B. *Forgive and Forget: Healing the Hurts We Don't Deserve.* San
Francisco: Harper & Row, 1984.

Sontag, Susan. *Illness as Metaphor.* New York: Farrar, Straus & Giroux,
1977.

Sourkes, Barbara M., Ph.D. *The Deepening Shade.* Pittsburgh: University of
Pittsburgh Press, 1982.

Swirsky, Joan, R.N., and Nannery, Diane Sackett. *Coping with Lymphedema.*
New York: Avery Publishing, 1998.

Toner, Robin, and Leslie Kaufman. "Ruling Upsets Advocates for the
Disabled." *New York Times,* June 24, 1999.

Tucker, M. A., M.D., et al. "Risk of Second Cancers After Treatment for
Hodgkin's Disease." *New England Journal of Medicine* 318 (1988): 76–81.

Veninga, Robert. *A Gift of Hope: How We Survive Our Tragedies.* Boston:
Little, Brown, 1985.

Viorst, Judith. *Necessary Losses.* New York: Ballantine, 1986.

Index

Late effects of treatment, 170n, 196
Laughter. *See* Humor
Laws. *See* Federal laws; State laws
Lazarus syndrome, 85–87
Legal action: against coworkers' os-
    tracism, 159; against insurance com-
    pany, 124–25; against job discrimina-
    tion, 156
Leigh, Susan, 196
Letting go, 96, 100
Leukemia, 34, 41–42, 51, 104, 105,
    119–20, 143, 210, 231–32
Leukemia Society, 104, 106
Leukeran, 211, 215
Lifestyle habits: and chronic fatigue, 185–
    87; diet and nutrition changes, 23, 68,
    69, 186; exercise, 68, 69, 181, 186; of
    inner peace, 68; meditation, 23, 68;
    and risk for secondary tumors, 189
Limb-salvage techniques, 172, 237
"Live for today" approach, 72, 74
Long-term effects of treatment. *See*
    Treatment long-term effects
Loss. *See* Grief
Lung fibrosis, 175
Lymphedema, 171, 178–84, 190, 200,
    232–33
Lymphoma, 39–41, 76, 79–81, 187

Mack, Connie, xiv
Magnetic resonance imaging (MRI), 64
Maintenance therapy, 37
Managed care programs, 109–10, 195–96
Manual Lymphatic Drainage (MLD),
    182–83
Marriage. *See* Divorce; Families; Fertility
    and infertility; Intimate relationships;
    Sexuality
Mastectomy, 21, 27–29, 31, 45, 54–55,
    90–91, 96, 118, 120, 188–89, 233
Mead, Margaret, 164
Mechlorethamine, 175, 215
Medicaid, 118–19, 137–38
Medical alert bracelet, 181

Medical examination. *See* Follow-up
    medical care; Physical examination
Medical Information Bureau (MIB), 108,
    136
Medical records for survivor, 36
Medicare, 121, 137–38
Meditation, 23, 68
Melanie, 71–72, 74
Melanoma, xiii–xvi
Melphalan, 187
Memory problems, 176–77, 192–93
Menopause, early, 188
Metastasis to lungs, 85
Metropolitan Life Insurance Company,
    143
Meyskens, Frank, Jr., 195
MIB (Medical Information Bureau), 108,
    136
MLD (Manual Lymphatic Drainage),
    182–83
Money management, 70
Monique, 31–32, 33, 34
MOPP, 213
Mourning. *See* Grief
MRI, 64
Mullan, Fitzhugh, 199, 237
Mustargen, 213, 215
Myelodysplastic syndrome, 187
Myleran, 211, 215
Myths about cancer, 141–43

Nader, Ralph, 132, 133
Nadia, 14–15
National Association of Claims Assis-
    tance Professionals, 137
National Association of Insurance Com-
    missioners (NAIC), 131, 137
National Breast Cancer Coalition,
    165–66
National Cancer Institute (NCI), xiii–
    xiv, 159, 198, 228
National Center for Chronic Disease
    Prevention and Health Promotion,
    168

Printed in the United States
109627LV00001B/95/A